ALL ABOUT CANCER
A Practical Guide to Cancer Care

ALL ABOUT CANCER
A Practical Guide to Cancer Care

Chris Williams

*Senior Lecturer and Honorary Consultant Physician,
CRC Medical Oncology Unit,
University of Southampton, UK*

A Wiley Medical Publication

JOHN WILEY & SONS

Chichester · New York · Brisbane · Toronto · Singapore

Library of Congress Cataloging in Publication Data:

Williams, Chris.
    All about cancer.

    (A Wiley medical publication)
    Includes index.
    1. Cancer. I. Title. II. Series.
RC263.W493   1983   616.99'4   82-13359
ISBN 0 471 90037 0 (paper)

British Library Cataloguing in Publication Data:

Williams, Chris.
    All about cancer.—(A Wiley medical publication)
    1. Cancer—Diagnosis   1. Cancer—Treatment
    I. Title
    616.99'4   RC270

    ISBN 0 471 90037 0

Typeset by Photo-Graphics, Honiton, Devon
Printed in Great Britain by Page Bros. (Norwich) Ltd.

To Saul Rosenberg and Gordon Hamilton Fairley

Acknowledgements

To my wife, Susan, for her help in 'humanizing' my efforts, her help in writing several sections, and proof reading. Virginia Souilah who steadfastly typed several drafts. Richard Hillier for his advice on several sections, and Peter Jack for his excellent illustrations.

I would also like to thank the following individuals and organizations for helping me by providing illustrations or reference material.

Duncan Ackery, Keith Dewbury, Peter Guyer, David Hands, Andrew Hayes, Susan Hubbard, Peter Isaacson, Suzie Miller, and Janice Middleton, Philips Medical Systems, Siemens Ltd., Toshiba Corporation, Wessex Cancer Trust, The Women's National Cancer Control Campaign.

Contents

Introduction

Cancer is not only a frightening disease – it is also surprisingly common. Most of us associate it with slow painful death even though many cancers can be cured and uncontrollable pain is rare. But the really frightening thing about cancer is the silence and 'taboo' that surrounds it. The sole aim of this book is to give plain, factual information about cancer, its diagnosis and treatment.

With this in mind the first chapters discuss what cancer is all about and what causes it. This is followed by sections on diagnosis of cancer and the treatment of individual tumours. The last part of the book is concerned with the treatment of symptoms and the emotional aspects of the disease. Hopefully this book will increase understanding of all aspects of cancer. It is intended for patients and their families, medical students and those working with cancer patients including family practitioners.

As well as the good news, if it is to be honest this book must contain much that is frankly depressing for the patient. Many doctors feel it their job to offer encouragement, even if this means distorting the truth or telling lies, but most people are more perceptive than one would imagine and this rarely allows a relationship of trust to develop. I therefore assume that anyone, patient or relative, picking up this book will be expecting truthful information.

Some patients with potentially serious illnesses visit the library to learn more about their disease. Though this can be helpful it is worth remembering that medical approaches, especially in cancer, are changing all the time and that a book more than five years old is probably out of date (and that includes this book).

It cannot be stressed too strongly that the best approach to the treatment of cancer should be to *care* for the patient as a human being and not just to treat the tumour. Previously most emphasis was put on getting rid of the tumour but nowadays there is equal appreciation of the importance of dealing with all the problems associated with cancer, whether it is curable or not. Facilities needed are not just new expensive equipment but more sophisticated caring arrangements such as mastectomy nurses to give advice and support and continuing care centres or hospices for the dying. These *should* be readily available to everyone wherever they live.

CHAPTER ONE

What is cancer?

To most of us cancer means certain death and we prefer to bury our heads in the sand about the subject, unless it affects us personally. Then we wonder what exactly has gone wrong and how did it start? It is a difficult question to answer but this chapter aims to give a simple explanation.

Normal tissues in the body are made up of individual building blocks or cells that can divide and multiply. This ability is controlled so that cell death and cell birth are roughly equal in an adult. In a cancer the control mechanisms that maintain this balance are lost and there is uncontrolled growth of cancer cells that exceeds the death of normal cells in that tissue. The tumour composed of the cancer cells continues to grow at the expense of the patient. It may invade local tissues, spread to nearby structures or even to distant organs. It is the invasion of local tumour or its distant spread that can cause symptoms or death. Cancer is, therefore, the uncontrolled growth of cells that will, if not stopped, spread locally, or to other parts of the body.

A cancer develops from a single cell following changes in the genetic material (DNA) with the cell. DNA carries the coded information that instructs the cell how to behave and an abnormality in the DNA may result in growth that does not respond to normal controls. If we cut ourselves the injured cells respond by dividing to repair the wound. Once repair has taken place the cells send out signals to neighbouring cells that instruct each other to stop multiplying. It is the failure to produce these signals or to respond to them that is the hallmark of cancer. The nature of these control mechanisms is one of the major unanswered questions in present day biology and until we explain the working of normal cell division and tissue growth it is unlikely that we will understand what is wrong in cancer and learn to restore normal control. The growth of normal cells and loss of normal control in cancer cells is shown diagrammatically in Figure 1.

A popular misconception about cancer is to think that it is one disease. Although, in each of the hundred or more types of cancer,

2

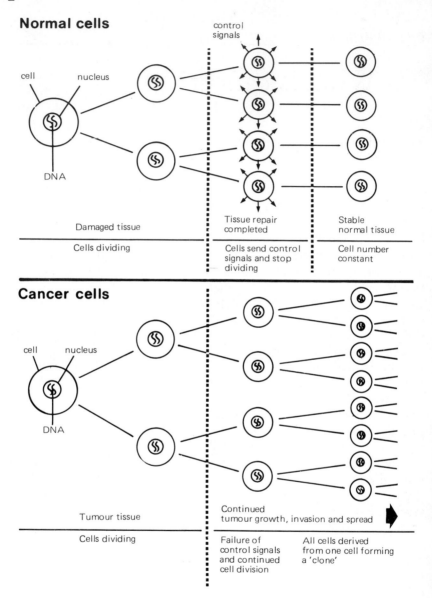

Figure 1 Diagrammatic representation showing the controlled growth of normal cells after injury to a tissue in comparison with the uncontrolled growth of cancer cells

cells have lost their controlling 'brake' the way that each tumour grows and spreads is individual. Because of the individual behaviour of each type of cancer the approach to treatment and its chance of success vary. Any generalizations about cancer are therefore best forgotten. Individual cancers can only be discussed in terms of a particular tumour type and at a particular stage of its spread.

It is my hope in this book to discuss, in a simple way, methods of diagnosing cancer, assessing its spread and finally how to treat it. As well as this factual information, emphasis will be placed on the problems associated with the fear of cancer, its treatment and ways of getting help with problems and anxieties that arise.

CHAPTER TWO

What causes cancer?

One of the commonest questions a patient with newly found cancer asks is 'Why have I got cancer; why me?'. At this stage most patients are more concerned with *why* the tumour has occurred, than what can be done about it. Usually it is just not possible to give a direct answer to this question as we still have so much to learn about the causes of cancer.

One thing to be said is that there are probably many causes and that more than one may be needed to produce each individual tumour. It is thought most cancers are caused by exposure to chemicals (called carcinogens: substances that can cause cancer). These carcinogenic chemicals are not necessarily man-made, but may be all round us in our natural environment.

Carcinogens affect cells by altering the normal DNA (DNA is the genetic material that controls cell function) in the centre or nucleus of the cell. Damage to the DNA can be repaired, may cause the cell to die or may produce no detectable change. Occasionally, however, it may cause a change which results in cancer.

Since finding out that certain substances or chemicals can cause cancer many others have also been identified or are suspected to be cancer causing because of their resemblence to known carcinogens. The problem is often a little more complicated than this as more than one carcinogen may be required to produce a cancer. If a chemical can be shown experimentally to cause cancer by itself it is described as a complete carcinogen. Other carcinogens (initiating factors) may produce changes in DNA which only result in a malignant tumour if the cell is exposed to a second substance (a promoting factor). It seems likely that this second type of mechanism is responsible for most human tumours and because of this more than one chemical or cancer causing agent is required to produce many types of cancer. Sorting our these carcinogens (whether complete or not) is a major problem. The first carcinogens to be described were discovered because of special exposure (usually in industry) to chemicals which caused unusual tumours that were easily recognized. For instance, the first demonstration of a carcinogenic substance was by Percival Pott in 1760 when he recognized that chimney sweeps had a very high incidence of cancer of the scrotum—because they were exposed to cancer-causing oils in soot which were rubbed into their clothes.

Although industrial exposure of groups of workers is very important and has taught scientists much about the way cancers are caused, the study of carcinogenic substances in our every-day environment remains a major problem. As we are all bound to be exposed to chemicals it is difficult to identify possible culprits. The problem is made more difficult as there are no obvious warning signs. Carcinogens act silently and frequently do not produce cancer for many years (an interval known as the latent period). After exposure to cancer causing substances this interval may be up to 20 years. Because of this we must try to identify carcinogens in the environment so that they may be removed (if possible) or ways of counteracting their effects be developed before a great number of people have been exposed to them for a long time.

Viruses have been shown to cause cancer in some animals but so far they have not been proven to cause human cancer. Despite this

Table 1 Estimated causes of human cancers	
Cause	Estimated proportion of cancer deaths in Western countries* (%)
Environmental	
Cigarette smoking	35
Diet	30
Occupation	2
Background radiation	2
Non-environmental	
Genetic	5
Total	74
Unaccounted for	26

*This estimate is based on figures from the United States.

it is likely that a few cancers in man are due to viruses, but do not worry that there may be an epidemic of cancer, a complex set of circumstances is probably needed before a cancer is caused by the virus.

There are other causes, some known (like radiation) and others unknown. Anyone worried about all the potential threats around them could drive themselves crazy if they made a list of all the *possibilities*. Maybe it is glue on envelopes, hair spray, sellotape, watching television, sucking a pencil, drinking coffee, infections in a swimming pool, or a thousand and one things we do every day. Clearly worrying about everything is fruitless, so if we are concerned about cancer it should be about the things we know of. Table 1 lists these and estimates the amount of influence that each factor exerts. It is obvious that the only factor easily changed is smoking.

CHAPTER THREE

How can we find cancer causing substances (carcinogens) in the environment?

A lot of research has gone into trying to find out about cancer producing agents and one way of doing this has been to see if people exposed to certain chemicals develop cancer. An example of this has been the finding of high incidence of tumours of the lining of the lungs in workers exposed to asbestos and this approach has been used to look at cancer in different countries.

In certain countries some tumours seem to occur often and in other countries hardly at all. This may be explained two ways. First, the high incidence of cancer may be due to an inherited predisposition to that tumour in the country of high incidence. An alternative explanation may be that the population in the high incidence country is exposed to carcinogens in their environment which are not present in the country with a low tumour incidence. Studies of the patterns of disease in various countries (epidemiology—the study of patterns and spread of diseases) has shown remarkable differences in the incidence of individual tumours around the world and it seems that the majority of the differences are best explained by local environmental factors and not by an inherited tendency to cancer.

The incidence of breast cancer in Japan, for instance, is much lower than in the Western world. However, when Japanese women move to Hawaii or the United States their incidence of breast cancer increases within one or two generations to resemble that of the non-Japanese population, even if they marry within their culture. Finding out which factors in the environment or diet cause this change is much more difficult as there are so many variations in life style and more than one may be blamed.

There has been some concern in the Western world that man-made chemicals can cause cancer and organizations such as the Federal Drug Administration (FDA) in the United States run tests on all new chemicals to see if they are carcinogenic. Much of the controversy over this screening has been about the types of test used and their interpretation. No test is ideal and it is just not possible to use tests in animals that mimic the long term exposure to low doses of chemicals that happens in man. Animals have a much shorter life-span, the tests take too long to complete and would be far too expensive. Instead, animal testing is usually done by giving very high doses of the chemical. Experts criticize the use of high doses of chemicals as the results may not be applicable to people exposed to much lower doses over a long period. It is all rather inconclusive and unsatisfactory.

The arguments recently surrounding saccharin (an artificial sweetener) show the difficulties of this approach. Rats were exposed to high doses of the drug and some developed bladder cancers and there were demands that saccharin should be taken out of the shops. However, critics argued that the results were meaningless and pointed out that the dose used was the equivalent of someone drinking about 800 cans of diet soft drink each day! Other experts argued that there was no safe dose for a carcinogen and they said that saccharin is used by millions and even low doses, if used over a long period, may result in thousands of extra cases of cancer. The question, therefore is unanswered, but many feel that any risk is unacceptable. Animal experiments designed to detect a very low incidence of cancer (though very important in the whole population—i.e. a chemical causing cancer in one in a thousand people each year would, if all the people in Britain were exposed, produce 60,000 new cases of cancer a year) are just not feasible, particularly if it is remembered that there are thousands of substances to test each year.

In an attempt to get around the problem of the large numbers of new chemicals to be tested each year initial screening of chemicals to see if they react with DNA (substances that do react with DNA are called mutagens) is now being used. These simple tests, which do not use animals, may pick up many potential carcinogens (though not *all* carcinogens may be mutagenic) which can then be tested in animals to see if they are cancer causing. But we still need a test for environmental carcinogens that is cheap, simple, quick, and accurate.

If we do find a carcinogen what can be done about it? Cigarettes are a good example. We all know cigarettes are harmful to health, they cause lung cancer and heart and blood vessel disease but stopping smoking is a hard thing to do, even for the most determined of us.

Both governments and manufacturers have a financial interest in keeping the habit going and it is often not until cancer or a heart attack strikes that the motivation is strong enough to stop smoking and really by then it is too late, the damage is done.

So accepting that there are problems in identifying cancer causing agents and restricting their use, what are the risks?

RISK AT WORK

We know most about cancer causing agents through the investigation of chemicals in the work-place. Many people are at risk from exposure to carcinogens, though the number of cancers which result is not known. A short list of potential carcinogens and the types of jobs where they are used is shown in Table 2. This table is not at all complete and only *some* of the workers in the industries mentioned are at risk—an idea of potential risk in a particular job can only be given by company or union doctors, and scientists. Ideally carcinogens should be completely banned but as this is not realistic strict precautions should be enforced in the face of recognized hazards, e.g. asbestos, though this is often not done. The problem with carcinogens is their lack of warning signs—a seemingly innocent substance may only cause cancer after a 20-year latent period. It is therefore difficult to persuade workers to observe safety precautions; especially when these may be inconvenient.

For those likely to be exposed to chemical carcinogens at work the only choice they have apart from changing jobs is to ensure that they protect themselves adequately by carrying out all the safety measures necessary. Safety is not only the responsibility of employers and unions but also of workers. There is also some evidence that workers exposed to carcinogens should not smoke as this may increase the risk of cancer and this is certainly true in the case of asbestos where the risk of cancer is far higher in those who also smoke.

10

Table 2 Carcinogens (chemicals which can cause cancer) in the work-place*

Agent	Job	Type of cancer
Non-organic		
Arsenic	Oil refineries, smelting, insecticide manufacture and spraying, tanneries and general chemical industry	Liver, skin and lung
Chromium	Glass and pottery manufacture, acetylene and analine industry, battery making, and bleach industry	Larynx (voice box), lung, and nasal passages
Iron oxide	Iron foundries, iron-ore mining, metal grinding and polishing	Larynx and lung
Nickel	Nickel smelting and electrolysis	Nasal passages and lung
Leather dust	Leather works and shoe-making	Nasal passages, bladder and urinary tract
Wood dust	Wood workers	Nasal passages
Asbestos	Insulation workers, shipyards, brake and clutch repairers, asbestos miners, and millers	Lung, pleura (lining of chest and lung), peritoneum (lining of the abdomen)

Organic substances		
Paraffin Petroleum Mineral oils Wax Shale Coke	Welding, workers in contact with lubricants, oils, paraffin	Lung, larynx, skin, scrotum
Coal soot Coal tar	Asphalt, coal tar, and pitch workers, gas works, chimney sweeps, coke oven workers, miners	Lung, larynx, skin, bladder
Benzene	Dyestuffs, painting, shoe-making, explosives, benzene manufacture, and adhesives	Leukaemia
Benzidine, α-naphthylamine, β-naphthylamine, 4-aminodiphenyl	Dyestuffs, rubber industry, textile dyeing and paint-makers	Bladder
Vinyl chloride	Plastic manufacturer	Liver and brain
bis (chloromethyl) ether, chloromethyl ether	Chemical workers	Lung
X-rays, uranium, radium, radon, plutonium	Atomic energy industry, x-ray personnel, chemists and researchers, miners (radon)	Skin, bone marrow (leukaemia), lung
Ultraviolet rays (sun)	Outdoor workers	Skin

*This list is not exhaustive and not all workers in the industries mentioned are automatically at risk from exposure to carcinogens.

ARE THERE RISKS APART FROM WORK?

It is only relatively recently that we have started to look for cancer causing substances and we have not discovered all the risks, though some definite and suspected carcinogens are present in our everyday environment.

Several colour additives have been taken off the market by the FDA (Federal Drug Administration) in the United States and many of the other additives have been suspected as they are similar to known carcinogens, the aromatic amines of coal tar (Table 2). Although very small quantities of these dyestuffs are present in each product they are very widely used in processed foods and consumption is therefore high over a long time period. No risk has been defined and it is not possible to check if there is any risk by our present screening methods (Page 8). There has also been controversy over the amounts of nitrates and nitrites which are present in preserved foods.

CHAPTER FOUR

Who is at high risk of getting cancer?

Those people most likely to develop cancer fall into one of several groups which are discussed in this section. Table 3 shows the degree of risk for various groups of people for the common tumours.

INHERITED CANCERS

There is absolutely no inherited risk of cancer for most people except for a very few in whom the tendency to develop the disease is greater for certain genetic reasons.

Cancer families

There are some rare families who have a very high incidence of certain cancers. The commonest cancers in these families are those of the large bowel, womb (uterus), stomach, and breast. The tumours tend to occur at an unusually early age and may develop in several places at once. These patients have a *very* strong family history (over several generations) of cancers and if this is part of your family pattern it is wise to be alert for symptoms and contact your family doctor if you are at all suspicious that there may be a problem.

Polyposis coli and Gardener's syndrome

These are inherited conditions in which there are many (often hundreds) of polyps in the large bowel. These polyps (fleshy outgrowths) are harmless but may become cancerous. Multiple polyps usually develop by the age of 20 and can be detected by a special x-ray, a barium enema (page 46). As the risk of cancer is very high in these conditions it is usually advised that the large bowel is removed (colectomy) before a tumour can develop. This

13

Table 3 Factors increasing the risk of developing some common cancers

	Lung	Breast	Uterus (womb)	Cervix (neck of womb)	Oesophagus (gullet)	Large Bowel (rectum and colon)
Moderate risk (2–3 times normal)	Smoking 5–9 cigarettes per day; family history in immediate relatives	Family history (immediate female relatives); possibly high fat diet; menopause after 52 years; obesity; first child after 30 years of age; no children	Family history (immediate female relatives); menopause after 52 years; moderately overweight; no children; medium doses of oestrogen drugs	Many sexual partners or early sexual intercourse (before 18 years)	Heavy alcohol consumption or smoking 20 cigarettes per day	Family history (immediate family); high fat and protein diet with low roughage
High risk (4 times greater or more)	Family history and smoking 1–9 cigarettes per day; smoking 10 or more cigarettes per day	Two or more of the above risk factors	Obesity; two or more of the above risk factors; high dose, long term oestrogen drugs	Both risk factors above	Both risk factors above	Both risk factors above; ulcerative colitis; polyposis coli or Gardener's syndrome

means having a colostomy (bringing the bowel to the surface of
the abdomen (page 327) and it is very difficult for a young person to
adjust to such an operation. However, the alternative is an almost
certain chance of bowel cancer by the age of 40 years. It must be
stressed that a colostomy is *not* required for the vast number of
people who have a few polyps in the large bowel and after taking
them out (using a sigmoidoscope or colonoscope (page 72)
patients will just be monitored with intermittent tests.

Ulcerative colitis

(Not an inherited condition). Patients who have chronic ulcerative
colitis have an increased risk of cancer of the large bowel and this
risk becomes very pronounced after the ulcerative colitis has been
active for 10 years. For those with long standing colitis
(inflammation of the bowel) it is usual to remove the large bowel
(colectomy) in order to avoid the increasing risk of cancer. A
colostomy (page 326) is usually performed (bowel brought up to
the abdominal wall) though in some cases surgeons argue that the
small bowel can be connected to the rectum. The rectum is then
examined *regularly* (by a sigmoidoscope—page 72) so that any sign
of cancer can be detected early. This approach is, however, not
accepted by many doctors as it still allows for a risk of cancer.

Stomach cancer

People with pernicious anaemia (an unusual blood disorder) have
an increased risk of developing stomach cancer. Some doctors
suggest routine check-ups for these patients though this is not of
any proven benefit.

Breast cancer

In Western societies breast cancer is very common and there may
be a familial tendency here. Those women whose immediate
female relatives have early breast cancer (before 45 years) or cancer
of both breasts, have a higher than usual risk of developing breast
cancer themselves. Although routine self-examination of the
breast is recommended for all women (Chapter Seven), those at
high risk because of their family history should be seen by their
doctor for a routine check-up from their early twenties. After the
age of 30 routine mammograms are *probably* advisable in those at

highest risk. Routine screening is still unproven in many cancers but there does seem to be an advantage in screening those at high risk. A woman whose mother developed breast cancer before the age of 40 years has a one in five chance of developing a similar tumour and if her mother also developed another tumour in the other breast, within 10 years, the risk rises to one in two. However, a woman whose mother first developed a tumour after her menopause has a much smaller risk. For those at highest risk an operation to remove the breast tissue (a subcutaneous mastectomy) and replace it with an implant can be done.

Skin cancer

The commonest reason for most types of skin cancer is excessive exposure to sunlight. However, there are several rare inherited causes of skin cancers. (1) Xeroderma pigmentosa is an inherited condition in which the skin is unable to repair the damage caused by sunlight and multiple cancers develop. Protective measures to reduce exposure to sunlight will reduce the risk of cancers. (2) Albinism. This is an inherited condition in which there is a total lack of pigment in the skin, hair, and iris of the eye. Such people are very sensitive to sunlight and have a high incidence of skin cancer and avoidance of sunlight reduces the risk of cancer. (3) Neurofibromatosis. This is a rare inherited condition in which there are soft fleshy skin tags, brownish patches all over the skin and outgrowths on some nerves. These areas may undergo a cancerous change in about one in every 14 patients with the condition. (4) Malignant melanoma (malignant mole). This is a tumour of the pigment cells in the skin. It starts when a mole changes its character, it either grows, darkens, or bleeds and it does occasionally run in families so there may be an inherited predisposition to the tumour. It is more common in caucasian people living in warm countries as it is caused by exposure to sunlight.

Eye tumours

Retinoblastoma. This is a rare cancer of the back of the eye (retina). It develops early in life and about half the cases are inherited. The inherited type often occurs in both eyes and in families with such a history, children should have a regular eye examination in childhood.

OCCUPATIONAL RISK OF CANCER

Some jobs carry a risk of cancer because they expose workers to cancer causing substances (carcinogens—see Chapters Two and Three). Employees often find it difficult to get information about the risks associated with their job, this is due to an inability to accurately define which jobs carry a risk of cancer and a reluctance on the part of employers to openly discuss the potential risks that they are exposed to. Even when the risks are known, however, workers frequently disregard safety procedures.

It is just not possible to avoid using many of the known carcinogens and we have yet to discover others. Companies are unwilling to act against carcinogens until they are forced to do so by overwhelming evidence and public pressure and many are reluctant to discuss the risks of individual jobs though some employers do answer such questions if they are asked directly; such information (from company and union doctors) should ideally be available to all employees at risk. Table 2 on page 10 outlines *some* of the jobs that carry an increased risk of cancer.

ENVIRONMENTAL CAUSES OF CANCER

Everyone is exposed to carcinogens (Chapter Two) every day of their life. Until more is known about these substances it is hard to advise on ways of avoiding them. In the United States doctors have drawn up suggested simple guide-lines for avoiding potential cancer causing foods.

- Avoid foods containing nitrites and nitrates—these are mainly preserved meats, e.g. bacon and other cured meats.

- Avoid colour additives as much as possible. This is often difficult as many foods contain them, and a sensible balance may have to be accepted. In some countries a further difficulty is the lack of a list of contents on food tins or packages.

- Avoid food wrapped in polyvinyl chloride (plastic wrapping) or at least unwrap it before storing.

- Wash insecticides off all fresh fruit and vegetables.

- Avoid artificial sweeteners if possible, e.g. saccharin.

These guide-lines are completely untested but if used *may* reduce exposure to some carcinogens and the risk of developing

cancer. More extensive discussion of ways of avoiding carcinogens can be found in books described in Appendix C.

LIFE STYLE

Some cancers may be related to life style and consequent exposure
to carcinogens.

Lung cancer

It is not necessary to dwell on the effects of cigarette smoking
beyond saying that it is the most important carcinogen that we
know of and many thousands of cases of lung cancer a year could
be avoided; this is in addition to the even greater risk of
cardiovascular disease.

Cervical cancer

The risk of developing cancer of the cervix (neck of the womb)
appears to be related to sexual intercourse. Cervical cancer is most
common in women who start having intercourse at an early age
and with many different partners. Cervical cancer *may* be caused
by a virus infecting the vagina and cervix though evidence is not
strong. This virus could be transmitted during sexual intercourse.
The introduction of Pap smears of the cervix has meant that many
more cervical cancers are picked up at an early stage or when the
condition is pre-malignant (page 160). Routine pelvic examinations
and a cervical Pap smear ought to be done in women from their
early twenties.

Skin cancer

As mentioned earlier most skin cancers are related to exposure to
sunlight. A golden sun tan is attractive but unfortunately, this
increases the risk of various types of skin cancer if exposure is
excessive. Modern ultraviolet solariums do not carry this risk if
they are properly supervised, but because they produce a tan they
may, however, encourage people to stay in the sun for long
periods.

Obesity

Over weight women have a higher risk of developing both breast and uterine (womb) cancer. Loss of weight may be helpful in reducing the incidence of these tumours. This increased risk is probably due to hormonal differences that occur with obesity.

OTHER POTENTIAL CAUSES OF CANCER

Testicular cancer

The only known predisposing cause of testicular cancer is failure of the testis to descend into the scrotum. The testes develop in the abdomen and move downwards, reaching the scrotum just before birth and if this fails to happen (an undescended testicle) the risk of cancer of the testis is increased fifty-fold. It has become usual to operate and bring the testis into the scrotum before the age of 5 years if it has not descended. This was thought to prevent cancer from developing but new information suggests that the damage is done and that cancer may still develop. Some surgeons now remove the abnormal testis (which usually does not work, anyway) in order to prevent the risk of a cancer developing. Men with one testis are sexually normal and can father children.

Although most patients with a undescended testicle do not develop cancer, surgery to bring the testis into the scrotum is the least that should be done, as a tumour developing within the abdomen will not cause symptoms till an advanced stage.

KNOWN RISK FACTORS

Table 3 (page 14) outlines some of the major risk factors for six common types of cancer.

CHAPTER FIVE

Which are the common cancers?

It depends on which part of the world you live in as to which cancers are most common, but the commonest cancers in Britain and the United States are also amongst the commonest in

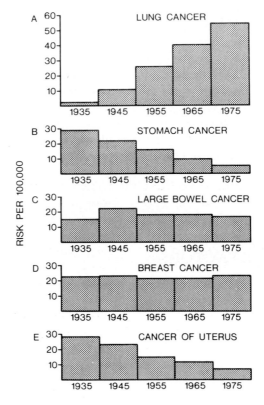

Figure 2 Changes in the frequency (expressed as cases per 100,000 population) for several common tumours during the years 1935–1975. Some become more common (especially lung) whilst others are seen less often

Table 4 Incidence of various common cancers, per 100,000 people, in
the United States* (adjusted for age)

Type (site) of tumour in order of frequency	Number of cancers/100,000 per year	
	Male	Female
Lung	70	13
Uterus	—	76
Breast	1	75
Colon	34	30
Prostate	59	—
Rectum	17	11
Bladder	22	6
Lymphomas	16	10
Stomach	16	7
Pancreas	12	7
Leukaemias	12	7
Mouth	11	4
Ovary	—	14
Nervous system	7	5
Kidney	8	4
Larynx	9	1
Oesophagus	6	2

*Although the exact incidence varies from country to country these data from
the United States are representative for most Western countries.

other Western countries. This may reflect an environmental cause
for many tumours.

The overall incidence of cancer, taking into account that people
are living longer, has not really increased in the past fifty years;
although some tumours have become more common and others
less common. The tumour that has increased most is lung cancer
whilst stomach cancer has become progressively less of a problem.
Figure 2 shows the changing pattern of occurrence for some of the
major tumours in the last fifty years and Table 4 the frequency of
the most important cancers.

CHAPTER SIX

Are there any warning signs of cancer?

An early diagnosis of cancer is very important. Most cancers grow from a single cell and may spread to other parts of the body. The smaller a tumour when it is discovered, the greater the chance that it has not spread. This means the patient with a small cancer is very likely to be cured by surgical removal of the tumour (see Chapters Nine and Twelve).

Noticing the possible warning signs of cancer is vital to picking up a tumour early. The following symptoms are a reason for consulting a doctor immediately. Ten false alarms are better than one delayed diagnosis. None of these symptoms automatically means cancer but a careful examination is needed to rule it out.

Many people dislike consulting their own doctor with seemingly trivial symptoms but they must be reported and no doctor will ever think that his time is being wasted. So make an appointment immediately if you have any of the following:

Breast Lump or thickening in breast, discharge from the nipple.

Colon and Rectum Change in bowel habit, rectal bleeding.

Lung Persistent cough, lingering chest infection, or coughing up blood.

Mouth, throat, and larynx (voice box) Sore that does not heal, difficulty in swallowing or change in voice.

Skin Sore that does not heal or change in wart or mole, bleeding from mole.

Uterus (womb) **and cervix** Any bleeding between normal periods or, after menopause, any bleeding at all, or any unusual discharge.

Kidney or bladder Pain or difficulty passing urine or blood in the urine.

Stomach Indigestion, difficulty in swallowing, or persistent vomiting.

The American Cancer Society has tried to improve the early diagnosis of cancer by bringing the common warning signs of cancer to the attention of the public. They use this mnemonic to warn of cancers anywhere in the body.

C hange in bowel or bladder habits.
A sore that does not heal.
U nusual bleeding or discharge.
T hickening or lump in the breast or elsewhere.
I ndigestion or difficulty in swallowing.
O bvious change in wart or mole.
N agging cough or hoarseness.

CHAPTER SEVEN

What is cancer screening?

If we accept that the treatment of cancer is most successful when a tumour is very small then it makes sense to try using special tests to detect tumours before they cause any symptoms. Cancer screening is a relatively recent idea and the assumption that it will improve the care of cancer remains unproven for many tumours.

Screening tests have been mainly concerned with a few common tumours and we will concentrate on these. Doctors do not all agree on the need for screening and trials testing the usefulness and assessing the cost and benefits of various types of screening are being carried out.

Most doctors in the United States recommend an annual general physical examination and though this is less accepted in Europe the potential role of such prophylactic medicine is attractive.

Cancer of the cervix (neck of the womb)

In many Western countries deaths from cervical cancer have been reduced by up to 50 per cent in the past 20 years. During this time there has been increasing awareness of the importance of early diagnosis and a concentrated effort to screen for the disease using the cervical smear technique or Pap test (page 72).

Cells from the cervix are examined under a microscope after they have been scraped from the lining of the cervix. Many of the cancers found by this method are localized to the surface and are called *in situ* cancers. Cervical cancer, when caught at this stage, is nearly always curable (more than 95 per cent). It is important to have routine smear tests done as tests performed when a woman has symptoms of cervical cancer are much more likely to show an invasive tumour which is more difficult to cure. In some women *pre*-malignant cells (cells that may turn into cancer cells) are seen and these women should have very regular screening to check if the smear is becoming more abnormal.

There are no universally accepted guide-lines on when the tests should be started and how often they should be done. Tests should probably be started at 25 years of age and be repeated annually, though some doctors will allow gaps of up to 3 years after two negative tests. Patients with abnormal vaginal bleeding or a persistent vaginal discharge should probably have a smear every 6 months for 2 years. Women with abnormal cells that may represent a pre-malignant change (called dysplasia) will need to have a biopsy of the cervix and, if available, direct microscopic examination of the cervix (colposcopy). If there is no sign of cancer they should be followed with further cervical smears at 6-monthly intervals.

Whilst the results of treatment of *in situ* cancers detected by smear are very good the smear has less impact when it picks up more advanced cervical cancer. The problem of this cancer is far from settled and even the role of mass screening is still being investigated. However, doctors agree that all women should have routine smears. The main problem with screening is that those women at greatest risk often do not come for the test.

Breast cancer

Breast cancer is the most common type of cancer in women living in the Western world. The breast is easily examined and there has been great interest in persuading women to undertake routine examination for breast lumps. This screening examination is of three types.

(1) The simplest is self-examination of the breast (Figure 3). Doctors should explain how this is done and recommend self-examination monthly. This is the first line of screening and a careful examination should pick up small lumps. Women still having their periods need to examine their breasts at the same time each month as the shape and feel of the breasts changes with the menstrual cycle. The best time to examine the breasts is 7 days after the start of each period.

(2) Breast examination by a doctor or specially trained nurse. This is usually done annually.

(3) Mammography. This is a special x-ray of the breast useful for detecting cancers too small to be felt. Although able to detect small tumours it also exposes the breast to irradiation

which can cause cancer itself. Though this risk is *very small* it must be balanced against the possible benefit of the test. Most doctors, for this reason, only recommend routine mammograms in patients over 50 years of age and possibly those at high risk. As improved mammography equipment, giving more accurate pictures and using a lower dose of irradiation (with less risk of cancer), become available it is likely that the mammograms will be used in younger patients for screening.

It is a pity but breast self-examination, is ignored by most women. Various 'Well Women' clinics have been set up around Britain which carry out routine regular screening programmes. Women should check if there is one in their area.

Although doctors are not agreed on the best ways to screen for breast cancer the following recommendations, represent current thinking in the United States and some European countries. The routine use of mammograms is less well established and is only available in screening studies in some countries.

(1) Women with no specific risk.
    Breast self-examination each month.
    Physical examination annually (this may be done at the same time as a Pap smear).
    Possibly mammography at age 50 and then periodically.
(2) Women with a positive family history of breast cancer.
    Breast self-examination monthly.
    Physical examination every 6 months.
    Possibly mammography at age 50 and then periodically.
(3) Women who have had a mastectomy previously.
    Breast self-examination monthly.
    Physical examination every 6 months.
    Possibly mammography annually.

All patients with a breast lump should be seen by a specialist so that it may be looked at closely and if necessary biopsied. The majority of breast lumps that are biopsied do not contain cancer (they are benign), but this can only be proved by examining the lump under a microscope. The decision, whether to perform a biopsy or not, can only be made by a specialist and general practitioners should refer all patients with a breast lump immediately to a breast clinic.

Inspection — How to look

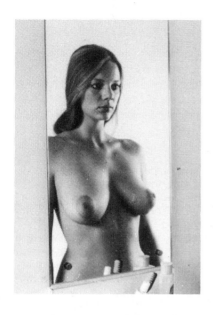

1. Undress to the waist and sit or stand in front of a mirror in a good light with your arms comfortably by your sides. If sitting, you may find it preferable to rest your hands lightly on your hips. Look at your breasts carefully. In the first examination you should note the normal size and shape of each breast and the position of the nipples so that you will be aware of any changes that might develop. In subsequent examinations you should look for any inequality in the size or shape of your breasts. Pay special attention to any alterations in the surface of the breast, such as a swelling, skin puckering (dimple), rash, discolouration or very prominent veins. Note whether either nipple is retracted (turned in).

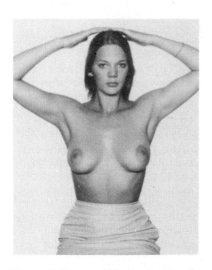

2. Now place the hands lightly on the top of the head and again look at the breasts carefully, concentrating especially on the nipples. This position will emphasize any difference in size or shape between the two breasts. Look particularly for any excessive upward or outward movement of either nipple.

Figure 3 Breast self-examination (reproduced, with permission, from a leaflet produced by The Women's National Cancer Control Campaign of 1 South Audley Street, London W1. International copyright of the Women's National Cancer Control Campaign)

28

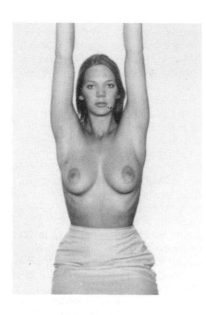

3. Momentarily stretch the arms above the head. Again this will emphasize any difference between the two breasts.

4. Now place the hands firmly on your hips and, when you are comfortable, push inwards towards the hips. You should feel the muscles on the upper part of your chest beneath your breasts tighten when you do this. Look at the breasts carefully while you keep pressing. This movement will emphasize any puckering of the skin or any abnormal retraction of either nipple. Remember to look at the under surface of the breast during this part of the examination. It is often easier to stand up to do this properly. You have completed the INSPECTION part of the examination and it is now time to feel for any abnormal lumps in the breasts. Again it is important at the first examination to note the normal consistency of your breasts, so that you will be aware of any change in subsequent examinations. Many women who have not yet reached the change of life normally have rather lumpy breasts just before the period and in some this may persist throughout the whole month. This may cause uncertainty at first, but with each successive examination it should become easier to decide whether any unusual lump is present.

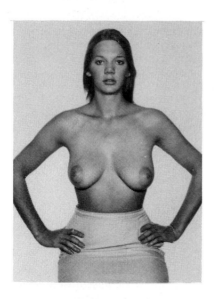

Figure 3 (*cont.*) Breast self-examination

Palpation — How to feel

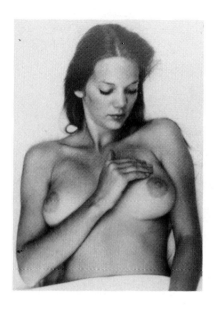

5. Lie down comfortably on a firm surface with your head on a pillow. Place a folded towel under the shoulder slightly raising the side that you are going to examine first. The left breast is felt with your right hand and vice versa. The first part of the examination is done with the arm by the side. Feel with the flat of the pads of the middle three fingers. The fingers should be kept straight but the hand flexible. Each time you feel, the breast tissue should be pressed towards the chest wall. Firm but gentle pressure should be used.

6. 7. 8. The examination starts just above the nipple and continues outward in a spiral fashion around the breast. EVERY PART of the breast must be felt so that two or three complete circles will need to be made depending on the size of the breast. Any unusual discrete lump or nodule should be noted.

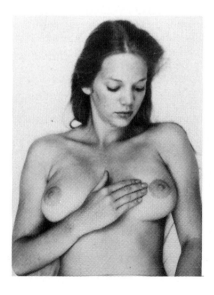

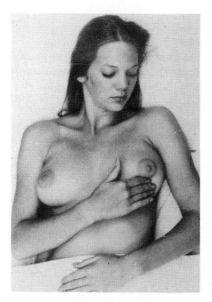 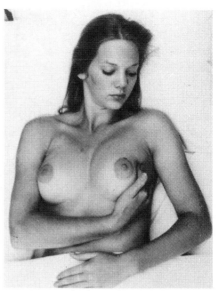

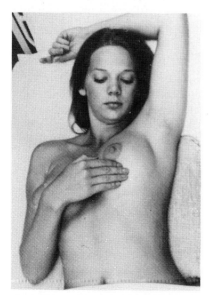

9. It is not easy to examine the outermost part of the breast with the arm by the side. When you have completed the first series of circular movements place the arm comfortably above the head with the elbow bent. Repeat the examination of all the breast now, paying especial attention to the outer part which can now be felt with more certainty. Never rush palpation of the breasts which must be done slowly, gently, and thoroughly.

Figure 3 (*cont.*) Breast self-examination

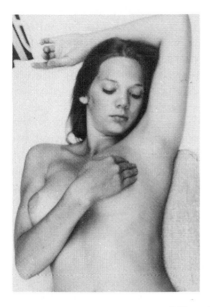

10. The final part of the examination is of the so-called tail of the breast which extends towards the armpit. This can only be examined properly with the arm above the head.

You have now completed palpation of one breast and this must be repeated for the other side.

Having completed self-examination of your breasts you will have decided whether they remain unchanged or whether any unusual feature has appeared. To remind you of these features, they are again listed below.

Warning Signs

ON INSPECTION

Unusual difference in size or shape of the breasts.

Alterations in the position of either nipple.

Retraction (turning in) of either nipple.

Puckering (dimple) of the skin surface.

Unusual rash on the breast or nipple.

Unusual prominence of the veins over either breast.

ON PALPATION

Unusual discrete lump or nodule in any part of either breast.

Routine Examinations

Try to make the examination of your breasts a monthly habit. Immediately following a period would be a suitable time, or on the first day of the month if you have had the menopause.

Cancer of the large bowel (Colon and rectum)

Screening for cancer of the large bowel is much more arguable. This tumour is common in the Western world and the outlook after surgical removal of the cancer is related to the extent of spread. Early diagnosis might, therefore, improve survival in this tumour. Most patients present with symptoms of constipation, diarrhoea, or rectal bleeding though harmless polyps may also cause similar symptoms.

Anyone with these symptoms should be investigated with a sigmoidoscopy, barium enema, and possibly a colonoscopy (see Chapter Eleven for explanation of these tests). If a harmless polyp is found in the colon this should be removed (using a snare through the colonoscope or sigmoidoscope) and routine follow-up examination can then be carried out every 2–3 years. Polyps grow slowly and some may slowly change to cancer; routine examination of the bowel will allow removal of any new polyps before they can become cancerous.

Nearly all cancers of the bowel bleed (90 per cent) and testing of the stools for blood (occult blood testing) is frequently used to screen for cancer. The place of occult blood tests and examination of the bowel using a sigmoidoscope or colonoscopy for screening is not clear. Many doctors in America recommend routine occult blood testing as it is simple, inexpensive, and rules out most cancers. Screening sigmoidoscopy or colonoscopy is not recommended by most doctors. However, patients with a strong family history of large bowel cancer or of one of the predisposing diseases (Chapter Four) should have regular screening tests.

Prostate cancer

Prostate cancer becomes more common after the age of 50 years. The prostate can be felt during a rectal examination and any abnormal lump or nodule detected. If a routine annual physical examination is done this should include a rectal examination.

Cancers of the mouth

Cancers of the mouth and throat can often be seen or felt. A routine dental visit (at least annually) should allow early detection of many of these tumours. Dentists, in addition to looking after a patient's teeth, will carefully examine the soft parts of their mouth.

Cancer of the uterus (womb)

Cancer of the uterus is not reliably diagnosed by a cervical or Pap smear. The only sure way to detect uterine cancer is by a D and C (D and C stands for dilatation and curettage, this is the scraping away of the lining of the uterus under general anaesthetic for microscopic examination) or by jet washings. These tests are expensive and can be uncomfortable, and if a D and C is done the patient needs to be admitted to hospital for a short period.

These tests are, therefore, not used to screen for cancer. Any abnormal vaginal bleeding is an indication for investigation and frequently a D and C is needed to be sure that there is no uterine cancer.

Lung cancer

Screening chest x-rays have not been shown to improve the survival chances of most patients with lung cancer. This is because lung cancer has usually spread before it can be seen on a routine chest x-ray. However, a chest x-ray should form part of any routine annual physical examination as it provides information about diseases other than lung cancer, though the advantages of routine examination remain unclear. Preferably doctors should recommend that patients stop smoking altogether.

Malignant melanoma

In Australia, where malignant melanoma is a very common skin cancer, special clinics for early diagnosis have been set up. Patients with skin lumps are encouraged to come to these clinics and tumours are being recognized at an earlier stage—when the chance for cure is greatest.

CHAPTER EIGHT

How is the diagnosis of cancer made?

Although a doctor may suspect cancer a diagnosis cannot be made without examining a piece of the suspicious tissue under a microscope. A biopsy (removal of a piece of tissue for examination — by a small operation or by a needle) **Must** be done if cancer is suspected. For details on how biopsies are performed see Chapter Twelve and the sections on each of the common tumours.

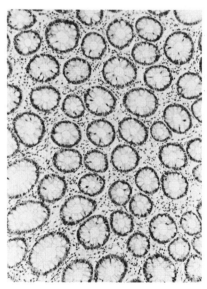

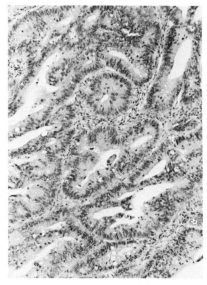

Figure 4(a) Normal stomach tissue: this microscopic view shows a regular appearance of symmetrical glands

Figure 4(b) Cancer of the stomach: this microscopic view (taken from the same patient as Figure 4(a)) shows that the glandular structure is grossly changed and that the cells making up the glands are different

When a biopsy has been taken the tissue is prepared and stained with special dyes for examination under a microscope. The doctor (a pathologist) looking at the biopsy will examine the pattern of the cells in the tissue and the characteristics of the individual cells (Figure 4). The pathologist will usually be certain if there is cancer and may be able to say where it has come from or if it has spread from somewhere else. Some types of cancer, however, may be difficult to detect and special tests may be needed on the biopsy or even another biopsy may be necessary to be sure of the diagnosis.

CHAPTER NINE

How does cancer spread?

One of the biggest problems doctors face in treating cancer is the spread of tumour (metastases or secondaries) to other areas of the body. Despite advances in surgical technique and anaesthetics, apparent complete surgical removal of a tumour is, in fact, often incomplete. Tumours frequently recur at the site they were taken away from, in nearby structures, or at other parts of the body.

Failure of surgery or radiotherapy to cure tumours is often due to spread of the cancer before treatment is ever started and an understanding of the ways that cancer spreads is clearly essential to planning treatment. Unfortunately our knowledge is limited; apart from a simple understanding of the routes of spread we do not know why or how each type of cancer spreads in the way it does. Table 5 shows the pattern of spread of the common tumours.

ROUTES OF SPREAD

Local invasion

Most tumours grow at the site where they originally developed. Some will invade nearby parts of the body and this may include spread of the cancer into major organs such as the bladder or bowel in the abdomen or into bones. Such invasion may cause pain, especially if the growth is into bone or local nerves and many of the early symptoms of cancer may be caused by this type of spread.

Lymphatic spread

The lymph system is a fine network of vessels, like blood vessels, whose job is to remove excess fluid and unwanted substances (including bacteria) from the body's tissues. If a tumour invades locally into these abundant lymph vessels it may spread via the vessels to nearby lymph nodes. Lymph nodes are pea-sized nodules scattered in various parts of the body. Their function is the filtering out of foreign material and the production of lymphocytes (a type of cell in the blood) which are part of the body's normal defences. The result is that lymph nodes trap the cancer cells in the lymph fluid and cancer grows within the node.

As there is usually a definite pattern of lymphatic drainage from most parts of the body doctors examine the draining lymph nodes for enlargement and the initial treatment plan may include therapy to these lymph nodes. Progressive spread along lymph vessels and nodes may occur so that quite distant nodes may become involved.

Distant spread by the bloodstream

If tumour invades blood vessels then cancer cells may break off into the bloodstream and be carried to other parts of the body. As blood vessels become progressively smaller these cells become trapped and the cancer may then develop at that point. The pattern of spread depends on the direction of the blood flow from the original tumour. The veins draining the bowel pass the blood on to the liver. Veins from the rest of the body drain into the heart and the blood then passes into the lungs. Thus the major site of spread in cases of bowel cancer is the liver. The lungs are the commonest site of metastases in other tumours though secondary liver involvement and spread to many other organs in the body are also common. The pattern of spread of individual tumours is discussed in the sections on the major types of tumours.

Risks and ways of avoiding recurrence of a tumour

(a) It is essential that there is a rim or margin of normal tissue surrounding a tumour when it is removed. If tumour is present in the margin around the lump removed then the cancer is likely to recur at that site. All surgical specimens should be examined to be sure that there is a tumour free margin.

(b) Lymph nodes draining the tumour should be examined by special x-rays or surgically. If there is evidence of spread to adjacent lymph nodes treatment for all the draining lymph nodes should be included in the initial treatment plan.

Table 5 Pattern of tumour spread for common cancers

Primary site of tumour	Risk of spread	Common sites of spread
Breast	★★★	Lymph nodes Bone Liver Lung
Lung	★★★	Lymph nodes Liver Bone, bone marrow Brain
Gastrointestinal tract		
Stomach	★★★	Local invasion Lymph nodes Liver Lung Bone
Pancreas	★★★	Local invasion Lymph nodes Liver Lung
Large bowel	★★	Local invasion Lymph nodes Liver
Gynaecological		
Ovary	★★★	Local spread and invasion Lymph nodes Liver
Uterus (womb)	★	Local invasion Lymph nodes Liver
Cervix	★★	Local invasion Lymph nodes

(c) Some tumours commonly spread by the blood to other parts of the body. Tests to see if spread has occurred should normally be done before therapy is started as the presence of secondary tumour (metastases) may alter the treatment plan.

Primary site of tumour	Risk of spread	Common sites of spread
Urological		
Kidney	★★	Local invasion Lymph nodes Bones Lung
Bladder	★★	Local invasion Lymph nodes
Prostate	★★★	Local invasion Lymph nodes Bone
Melanoma	★★	Local invasion and skin Lymph nodes Liver Lung Brain
Head and neck	★ or ★★	Local invasion Lymph node Lung
Lymphomas		
Hodgkin's disease	★★★	Lymph nodes Spleen Liver Lungs Bone/bone marrow
Non-Hodgkin's lymphoma	★★★	Lymph nodes Liver Bone/bone marrow Brain Lungs

CHAPTER TEN

What is staging?

When the diagnosis of cancer has been made it is important to know if the cancer has spread (see Chapter Nine) before
treatment can be planned. This is called 'staging' as the degree of
spread of a tumour is often referred to, by doctors, as the 'stage'
which it has reached.

The importance of staging lies in the different types of
treatment available. Both surgery and radiotherapy are 'local'
treatments. They are most effective when the tumour has not
spread beyond the local tissues where it arose. They may be used
successfully when there has been spread to draining lymph nodes
(see page 36) though the risk of unrecognized distant spread is
higher. Drug therapy (chemotherapy) is the mainstay of treatment
when the tumour is widespread. Accurate staging is important in
choosing the most effective treatment and also for avoiding
unnecessary therapy. Patients with metastatic disease (distant
spread) can be saved from extensive surgery or radiotherapy that
would not be useful.

The main aims of staging are to estimate:

(a) How large is the original tumour? Does it invade into
surrounding normal tissues?
(b) Has the tumour spread to nearby draining lymph nodes?
(c) Is there evidence of spread of cancer to other parts of the
body (metastases)?

The tests used to stage different tumours vary enormously. A
brief discussion of the types of tests carried out for the common
cancers are included in the sections on individual tumours and
details of the way the major tests are carried out are given in
Chapter Eleven.

For many tumour types there are special **staging classifications** that are used to describe the extent of spread of that
particular tumour. These are discussed in some of the sections on
the individual tumours.

Investigations used to diagnose and stage cancer

The major problem that doctors face when examining a patient is the inability to see what is actually going on inside the body. By taking an accurate detailed history, feeling (palpation), listening with a stethoscope, and testing the body's functions (i.e. testing reflexes) a physician gains information that helps make a diagnosis. Over the last fifty years a new branch of medicine has grown up that uses special tests designed to examine the inside of the body. Tests that will outline and show the extent of spread of a tumour are clearly of major importance and all patients with cancer will have some of the tests discussed in this section. The type and number of investigations will depend upon where the tumour started to grow (Chapters Nine and Ten) and this section outlines some of the commoner investigations. It is important that patients ask their doctor about the individual tests before they are done as there may be variations in technique from hospital to hospital. Tests not included here will need to be discussed and a list of suggested questions is included at the end of the chapter.

RADIOLOGY

This is the use of x-rays to produce a photographic film which outlines the body's tissues by their density. Dense tissues (e.g. bone) absorb more x-rays than less dense structures, such as lung, and an outline of the organs by their density (Figure 5) is produced on an x-ray plate (a photographic negative). This is the basis of conventional x-rays, such as a routine chest x-ray, that most people are familiar with.

Radiological tests can be divided into two broad categories:

(1) Plain films.
(2) Contrast studies.

41

42

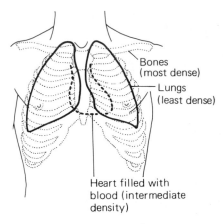

Figure 5(a) Diagrammatic representation of the structures of the chest as they show up on an x-ray. Bone is most dense, then the heart, and the lungs are least dense

Bones (most dense)

Lungs (least dense)

Heart filled with blood (intermediate density)

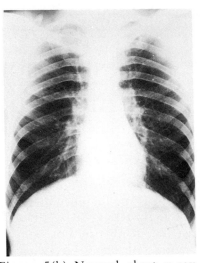

Figure 5(b) Normal chest x-ray showing how the bones, heart, and lungs are seen according to their density. The heart is dense (white) and shows up most clearly because it is so much bigger than the bones even though they are more dense. The lungs are hardly seen (very dark) as they are filled with air

Plain films are ordinary x-rays taken of any part of the body without special preparation or procedures. Examples are the routine chest x-ray or bone x-ray that we are all familiar with. Plain films or x-rays are of less use in examining many other parts of the body. This is because the consistency (density) of the various parts of the body are similar, and special ways to increase the density of an organ being examined are needed. Dyes or *contrast media* which are dense and show up clearly on x-rays are given so that the density of the structure is increased compared with the neighbouring structures (Figure 6).

The rest of this section outlines the various types of radiological tests, how they are performed, whether preparation is required, and discusses possible side-effects.

43

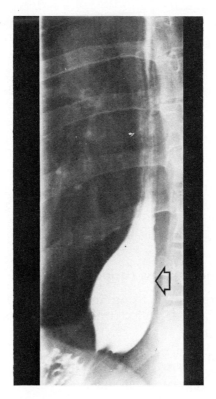

Figure 6 Barium dye outlining (see arrow) the oesophagus (gullet) in the chest

(a) Plain x-rays

These x-rays require no special preparation, are painless, and have no significant side-effects. In addition most x-ray departments do not need to book plain x-rays and are able to perform the test immediately. The time required for such x-rays is minimal.

All types of radiation including x-rays carry a *very small* risk of causing cancer themselves. At the doses used for routine x-rays, this risk is so small as to be meaningless. However, x-rays during pregnancy should be avoided, as the risks to a baby in the womb are higher. Tomograms (see page 57) are a special form of plain x-ray and are discussed separately.

Mammograms

- Mammograms are special plain x-rays of the breast. No special preparation is needed but talcum powder, deodorant, perfumes, or creams should not be used on the breasts for at least 24 hours before the tests as they cause shadows on the x-ray film.
- Women strip to the waist and the breast to be x-rayed is placed on a small platform and a cone shaped device gently compresses the breast. An x-ray of both breasts is usually taken. The test takes less than one hour and afterwards patients can carry on all normal activities.

(b) Contrast x-rays

Barium meal or swallow (upper G.I. series)

This is an investigation using *contrast material* (a barium compound) to outline the gullet (oesophagus), stomach, and upper part of the intestines.

- Patients are usually asked not to eat or drink for about 6 hours before the test and those patients taking regular drugs by mouth should check with their doctor.
- This test consists of drinking up to a glassful of a white cream (the barium mixture). Some people find the taste of this unpleasant. As the barium is swallowed, the radiologist (specialist in x-ray diagnosis), is able to follow its passage into the stomach and the upper digestive system on an x-ray screen (in a darkened room). X-ray films will be taken during the examination (Figure 7) and the series of films required usually means that the patient is tipped, on a mobile couch, into various positions so that the best views may be obtained. These include films lying in an upright position (on the couch) as well as films lying sideways.
- If only the gullet (oesophagus) is to be examined (barium swallow) the test should take less than half an hour. If a full barium meal examination is done, then the test is usually completed within 1½ hours. However, follow-up films the same day or occasionally on the following day may be needed in some cases. A barium meal and follow-through (an examination

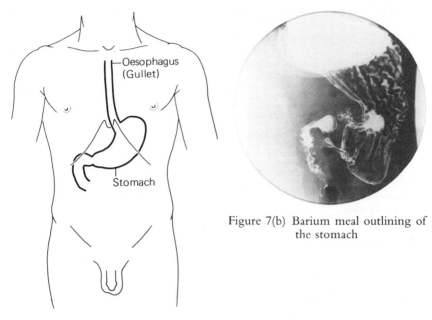

Figure 7(a) Diagrammatic representation of the upper part of the gastro-intestinal tract

Figure 7(b) Barium meal outlining of the stomach

of the stomach and small intestine) normally requires further x-ray films for at least 6 hours and possibly longer.

- Following a barium meal bowel motions may be affected, constipation and the passage of pale stools being the most common effect. Constipation is more common in people who are also using medicines for pain. A laxative may be given after the test.

- Many patients are able to drive home after a barium meal, but some feel a bit weak after the examination, particularly if they are obviously unwell before the test, and they will require help travelling home. The major discomforts of the test are drinking the barium which some patients dislike, and the tipping of the couch to obtain the best views.

Table 6 Minimal residual diet

Type of food	Foods included	Foods excluded
Drinks	Black coffee, tea, fizzy drinks	Milk, milk drinks
Bread	Dry biscuits	All breads
Desserts	Sorbets, clear gelatin, jelly	Custards, puddings, desserts made with milk, ice-cream
Fats	Bacon, butter	Cream
Meat, poultry, fish, cheese, and eggs	Lamb, veal, chicken, turkey, whitefish, eggs	Fried meat, poultry, or fish. All cheese
Potato, pasta	Macaroni, noodles, rice, spaghetti	Potatoes
Soups	Clear soups or broths	Cream soups
Vegetables	Tomato juice only	All vegetables
Condiments and spices	Salt, small amounts of pepper	All other spices, pickles, nuts, and olives

Barium enema

A barium enema is a special x-ray of the lower or large bowel (*colon* and *rectum*). To prepare for this, the bowel must be absolutely clean.

● Preparation for this x-ray will vary from hospital to hospital, but basically consists of:

(1) Eating a light diet for 2 days before the examination, e.g. meals of egg, but *not* meat, fish, fruit, or vegetables in any form. Patients should have plenty to drink. Table 6 shows the foods that may be eaten with a light or 'minimal residue' diet.
(2) A laxative is usually given to be taken the day before the test.
(3) Extra liquids should be drunk the day before the test and no solid food taken from the evening before the x-ray. A typical clear liquid diet is shown in table 7. No food or drink should be taken on the morning of the investigation.

Table 7 Clear liquid diet	
Type of food	Foods included
Drinks	Coffee, tea, fizzy drinks
Desserts	Sorbets, gelatin, jelly
Fruits	Fruit juices only
Soups	Clear soups, consommé, clear broth
Condiments	Salt

- Diabetics should not follow these instructions but should contact the doctor who is to perform the test and explain that they are diabetic. Alternative methods of preparation will be arranged.
- Before the barium enema can be done it is usual to wash the bowel out (an enema) to make sure that it is as clean as possible. After a variable period a barium mixture is run into the bowel by a tube passed into the rectum. The barium shows up on an x-ray screen (the room is darkened so the radiologist can see the screen clearly) and an outline of the large bowel can be recorded on an x-ray plate (Figure 8). These days it is common to pass some air into the lower bowel to distend it. The results of x-rays of the bowel by this method (called a double contrast barium enema) are usually much better than the old barium enema, without the air, and can pick up small abnormalities — cancerous or otherwise. When the barium and air have filled the bowel it will cause a sensation of pressure but it is important that the barium is held in the bowel till the x-rays have been finished.
- During the x-ray the patient may be turned or tipped (on a couch) to various positions to get the best x-ray view of different parts of the large bowel.
- The test takes up to 2½ hours including time for the wash-out of the bowel.
- The main problems with the test are the unpleasantness of the bowel wash-out and infusion of the barium and air.

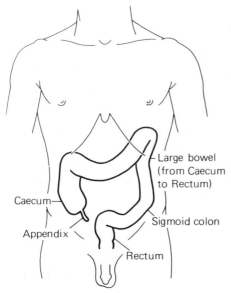

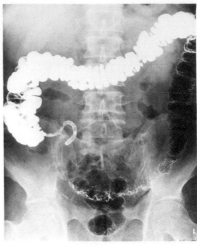

Figure 8(b) Barium enema outlining the large bowel

Figure 8(a) Diagrammatic representation of the lower part of the gastro-intestinal tract

- Many patients do not feel like driving after the test as it may be tiring, particularly for patients who are feeling unwell or weak before the examination.
- Patients will of course pass pale stools with barium in them for some days after the test. A laxative may be prescribed in order to remove the barium as quickly as possible.

Intravenous Pyelogram (IVP)

An IVP is a contrast x-ray to outline the *kidneys, ureters* (tubes connecting the kidneys to the bladder), and the bladder itself.

- To obtain the best view of the kidneys it is important that the overlying bowel should be cleaned out. Most hospitals therefore ask patients to take laxatives for 2 days before the test and to have a light meal the day before the test. On the day of the test patients will be asked **not** to eat **or** drink. Diabetics should tell the doctor arranging the test so that an appropriate diet can

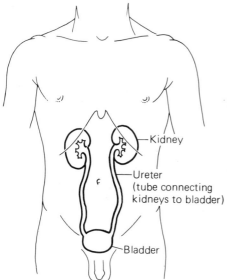

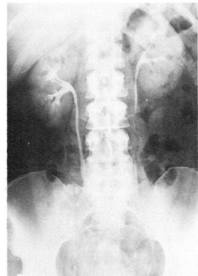

Figure 9(a) Diagrammatic representation of the kidneys, ureters, and bladder

Figure 9(b) Intravenous pyelogram showing dye outlining these structures

be arranged. Patients taking regular medicines by mouth should also check with their doctor.

- The technique of the test is to inject an x-ray contrast liquid into a vein in the forearm. This material will first appear in the kidneys and then outline the ureters and bladder (Figure 9). During the injection many patients feel hot and flushed and may be uncomfortable but this rapidly settles.
- Rarely patients may react against the dye (a type of allergic reaction). Patients becoming short of breath or feeling faint should tell the doctor giving the injection. If it is caused by a reaction this can rapidly be reversed by the use of simple drugs.
- Following the injection of the dye a series of x-rays of the abdomen are taken starting within 5 minutes and continuing for up to 1 hour.
- Occasionally a tight binder (about 25cm wide) is placed across the abdomen to improve the x-ray view.
- It is sometimes necessary to take late x-ray pictures if the doctor

wishes to follow the progress of dye through a kidney which is slow to pass the dye.

- Occasionally it may be necessary to perform tomogram x-rays (page 57)of a kidney to get the best view.
- The test usually lasts less than 1 hour and many patients are able to drive home afterwards though some may not feel very happy about this if the injection caused much flushing or discomfort.

Oral cholecystogram (gall-bladder series)

An oral cholecystogram is an x-ray taken to outline the *gall-bladder* after a contrast dye has been taken by mouth.

- As with most x-rays of abdominal organs it is necessary to clean out the bowel to get the best views. Laxatives are usually given for the two nights before the test. Following a light meal plain x-rays of the abdomen are taken and if these are satisfactory (the bowel is sufficiently clear) the patient will be given x-ray dye tablets to be taken at a specified time before the second part of the test.
- The patient will be asked to have a light breakfast (these foods are permitted; fresh vegetables — cooked without fat, fruit, lean meat, dry toast or bread, tea or coffee). The following foods must be avoided; milk, butter, cream, eggs, salad dressings, or any dairy product or foods containing fats. The tablets should be taken with water at the specified time and then *nothing* eaten though water may be drunk.
- The dye in the capsules is absorbed from the stomach and is then concentrated by the liver and passes into the gall-bladder which acts as a reservoir for the bile (Figure 10).
- The dye in the gall-bladder shows up on x-rays of the abdomen and outlines it. X-rays at varying times and in differing positions are taken to get the best view of the gall-bladder.
- It is sometimes necessary to ask patients to drink a little milk. This causes the gall-bladder to contract and squeezes the dye and bile into the tube (bile duct) connecting the gall-bladder to the bowel. It is to prevent this contraction that fatty foods must be avoided before the test.
- The test is frequently completed within 1½ hours though late films may be required in some patients.

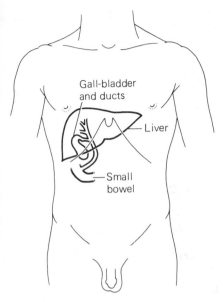

Figure 10(a) Diagrammatic representation of the relationship between the
liver, gall-bladder, and small bowel

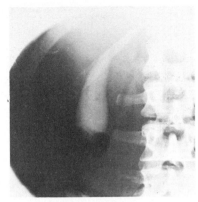

Figure 10(b) Cholecystogram
showing dye outlining the gall-bladder

- Most patients should be able to drive after the test and there is
no discomfort and no after-effects.

Lymphangiogram

A lymphangiogram is an x-ray examination of the *lymph vessels*
and *lymph nodes* of the legs and abdomen. The lymph system
consists of fine vessels, like blood vessels, which connect the
lymph nodes or glands. Their function is the removal of fluid or
unwanted substances in the body's tissues. The test is in two parts
spread over 2 days.

- *Day 1.* First of all the feet must be cleaned. The next part of the
test (Figure 11) consists of an injection (with a small needle) of
greeny-blue dye between the first and second toes of each foot.
This dye is taken up by the fine lymph vessels over the top of
each foot. Local anaesthetic is then injected to 'freeze' the skin.

52

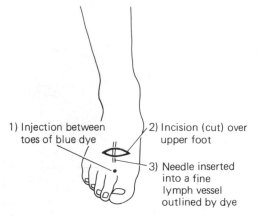

1) Injection between toes of blue dye

2) Incision (cut) over upper foot

3) Needle inserted into a fine lymph vessel outlined by dye

Figure 11 The technique used for a lympangiogram: (1) An injection of blue dye is given between the toes, (2) When the dye has been taken up by the fine lymphatics a small incision (cut) is made over the top of the foot, (3) A fine needle is then inserted into a tiny lymph vessel and dye injected

When this has taken effect the foot is cleaned again with alcohol and a small cut is made over the top of the foot and the fine lymph vessels (now outlined by the green-blue dye) are identified. A very fine needle is passed into a lymph vessel and a similar procedure is carried out on the other foot. A dye that shows up on x-ray (a radio-opaque dye) is then slowly injected under slight pressure so that it fills the lymph vessels in the legs and abdomen (Figure 12). This part of the procedure is tedious and takes about 2 hours and it is a good idea for patients to take along a book or magazine. Occasional check films to follow the progress of the dye will be taken. Skin stitches will be put into the cut on the top of the foot at the end of the test after the needles have been removed. A dry dressing is then put on the top of each foot.

- The test takes up to 4 hours and discomfort and tedium caused by lying still on the firm x-ray couch may be troublesome for some patients.
- The blue-green dye is passed out in the urine which is green for some hours. Some patients complexion may become slightly greenish so that they look 'grey' and unwell. Some patients may have 'flu-like' symptoms.

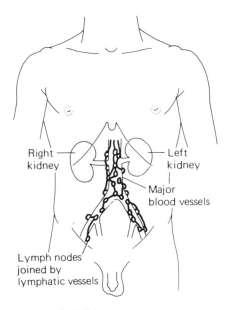

Figure 12(a) Diagrammatic representation of the lymph nodes at the back
of the abdomen

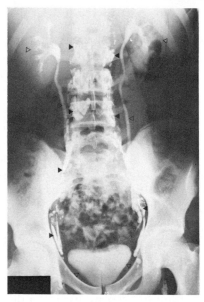

Figure 12(b) Lymphangiogram
showing dye outlining the lymph
nodes (closed arrows). The open
arrows show the kidney, ureters, and
bladder outlined by an IVP (page 48).

- Occasional 'allergic reactions' to the blue-green dye or x-ray
  contrast dye may occur. If patients are breathless or feel faint
  they should tell the doctor performing the test as the reaction
  can easily be reversed with simple drugs.
- Patients should sit with their legs raised as much as possible for
  the following 24 hours. This will stop their legs from swelling.
- Patients should not drive after this long examination as many
  will not feel up to it and driving may cause swelling of the feet.
- Patients should not allow their feet to become wet for at least 24
  hours, in order to avoid infection.
- *Day 2.* The next day a further series of x-rays of the abdomen
  and frequently an IVP (see page 48 will be done. Although
  there is usually no special preparation of the bowel, patients are
  often asked not to eat anything beforehand so that the best
  quality x-rays and IVP examination can be achieved.

- This part of the test lasts about 1 hour.
- Many patients do not like driving after the IVP (page 48) which often causes a temporary feeling of heat and flushing.
- The skin stitches in the feet should be removed 7–10 days after the test. A blue-green stain at the site of the injection on the top of the foot may persist for weeks and occasionally months.
- Soreness and swelling over the top of the foot are not uncommon and it is useful for the doctor to give the patient pain-killing tablets for the first few days after the test. Infection of the cut on the foot can happen and if the site of the stitches becomes very sore, inflamed, or discharges pus patients should see their own doctor. There are no other long term effects though doctors will usually avoid this test in patients whose lungs work poorly (such as in those with chronic bronchitis and emphysema) as some of the dye reaches the lungs and may *temporarily* reduce the lungs ability to work normally.

Arteriogram or Venogram

These are specialist tests used to outline an artery (arteriogram) or a vein (Figure 13). It is beyond the scope of this book to describe the techniques used for the different types of these tests as the method depends upon the site of the blood vessel being outlined.

- Briefly, it is necessary to place a fine plastic tube (a catheter) into the blood vessel to be outlined. This requires a minor operation which is usually done under local anaesthetic. If the test does require a general anaesthetic patients must not eat or drink for 6 hours before the anaesthetic. The technique needed to put the catheter into the blood vessel depends upon its site and should be discussed by the radiologist. In order to show up the vein or artery contrast dye is quickly injected and a rapid series of x-rays taken following it through the blood circulation of the area under investigation.
- During the injection of the dye patients may feel hot and uncomfortable although this feeling goes away quickly.
- The length of time it takes to do these tests depends on the blood vessel being investigated though most tests should take less than 2 hours.
- Most patients will not feel like driving after such a test. A small cut may be necessary to identify a blood vessel through which

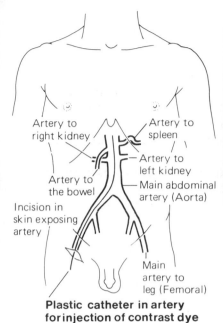

Artery to
right kidney

Artery to
spleen

Artery to
left kidney

Artery to
the bowel

Main abdominal
artery (Aorta)

Incision in
skin exposing
artery

Main
artery to
leg (Femoral)

**Plastic catheter in artery
for injection of contrast dye**

Figure 13(a) Diagrammatic representation of an arteriogram. In this case a
plastic tube (catheter) has been introduced into the artery in the groin and
fed up to the arteries in the abdomen.
An x-ray dye is then injected to show
up the blood vessels

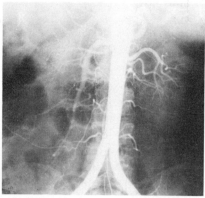

Figure 13(b) An arteriogram outlining
these blood vessels

the catheter is passed. This cut may be at some distance from
the vessel being tested as it is often not possible to get at the
blood vessel directly. For instance it is common to use the
blood vessels in the groin (femoral artery or vein) to get to
blood vessels in the abdomen (Figure 13). If a cut is made the
stitches will need to be removed about 7 days later.

- As with all tests using an injection of contrast dye, patients may
  very occasionally be allergic to the dye and patients becoming
  short of breath or feeling faint should tell the radiologist.
  Allergic reactions can easily be treated with simple drugs.
- There are usually no late complications though some bruising
  or discomfort where the catheter is put into the vein or artery is
  not uncommon. This should only last a few days.

These tests are often very specialized and the full details of the x-ray should be discussed with the radiologist.

Myelogram

A myelogram is an x-ray used to outline the *spinal canal* (the space around the spinal cord within the bony spine).

Under local anaesthetic a thin needle is passed between the bony vertebra in the lower back. The needle is then put into the fluid in the spinal canal (CSF) as in a lumbar puncture. This initial part of the test is identical to a lumbar puncture and some fluid is usually withdrawn for laboratory tests. Contrast dye which shows up on an x-ray of the back can then be injected into the fluid in the spinal canal. If the patient is tipped this heavy dye flows down the canal to show if it is completely open the length of the spine. Any restriction (partial or complete) will show up. If an obstruction is complete (dye cannot flow past it) and the radiologist (usually a specialist in neurological x-rays) wants to show the length of the obstruction he may also put a needle into the spinal cord at the top of the spine. This allows dye to flow downwards to the restriction and will show the upper level of the blockage. Most myelograms do not require this extra procedure.

- This test should be relatively painless though there is some discomfort when the initial lumbar puncture is done.
- Special preparation is not required.
- The length of time needed for the test depends partly on the findings, but is usually less than 1 hour.
- Many patients having this test will be in-hospital patients and they will be asked to lie flat for some hours after the test to reduce the risk of headaches.
- There should be no long term effects associated with the test. Some patients have a headache; this will improve on lying flat. Some radiologists remove most of the dye (depending on the type used) at the end of the test, as it may stay in the spinal canal and interfere with future x-rays of the chest or abdomen.

Other specialized contrast tests

There are other special x-rays, such as an air encephalogram, which are uncommon and beyond the scope of this book. The

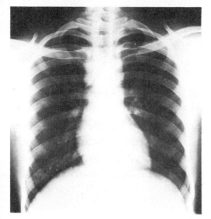

Figure 14(a) Chest x-ray which is relatively normal

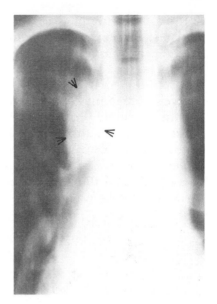

Figure 14(b) Close-up of a tomogram of the lungs of the same patient showing (see arrows) that the area around the heart (called the mediastinum) is wider than normal because of enlarged glands

doctor should take time to explain any test and the following points should be answered:

- What is the test for and how is it done?
- Is it uncomfortable?
- How long does it take?
- Are there any risks or side-effects?
- How will I feel after the test, can I go home, will I need someone to collect me; or will I be all right on my own?

Tomograms

Tomography is a special type of plain x-ray designed to get a better view of various parts of the body. When any x-ray is taken the film produced is made up of all the body's structures in front of the x-ray plate. In order to make unwanted structures blurred, whilst keeping the area being examined in focus, the x-ray machine is swung in an arc over the patient. The image of structures about which the x-ray machine pivots stay in focus whilst those in front or behind will be blurred. Small abnormalities (which may not be seen in an ordinary x-ray) can then be seen more clearly (Figure 14). A series of x-rays (known as cuts) of different parts of the area being examined are taken. After each x-ray the film plate underneath the table will need to be changed.

The length of time the test takes will depend on the number of cuts required. A full test may take an hour and may sometimes be used with a contrast study.

- No special preparation is required.
- The test is, of course, painless and has no side-effects.
- Patients should be able to see themselves home afterwards.

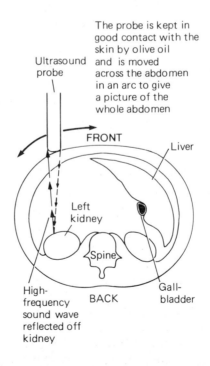

Figure 15 The basic theory behind ultrasound tests (see text for explanation)

ULTRASOUND (ULTRASONIC) TESTS

Rather than x-rays very high frequency sound waves are used for these tests. The frequency of the sound is far above that which the human ear can hear. A source of ultrasound waves is pressed against the body and a beam of sound waves is sent into the body. These waves strike areas of different density and sound waves are bounced back rather like the ASDIC system used to detect submarines (Figure 15).

- When the test is done on patients a probe looking rather like a microphone is used for the test. The probe must be in good contact with the skin and this is sometimes ensured by coating the skin with oil. The probe is then moved in an arc over the skin and it sends out and detects the reflected sound; the information is used to build up a picture of the area being examined (Figure 16). This is displayed on a television screen, and when the picture is complete an instant (polaroid) picture is taken for a permanent record.
- No special preparation is required. However, if the gall-bladder (page 50) is to be examined, patients will be asked not to eat anything for 6 hours beforehand, and if the lower abdomen or pelvis is to be shown, patients will be asked to come for the test with a **full** bladder.
- The test is entirely painless and ultrasound has no side-effects.
- Patients will suffer no effects from the test and may drive immediately.

CT BODY SCAN (also known as CAT scan, whole body scan, or body scanner)

This is a revolutionary new method of taking x-rays. This technique differs from a normal x-ray in two ways. First there is no normal x-ray film; instead there is an electronic x-ray detector. The second major difference is that both the x-ray source (equivalent to the old x-ray machine) and sometimes the detector rotate around the patient (Figure 17). The x-ray scanner produces a narrow beam of x-rays and as this rotates around the part of the body being examined, the detector receives information on the density or consistency of the body at that point. When the scanner and detector have rotated around the body, the information from all angles is processed by a computer which produces a picture

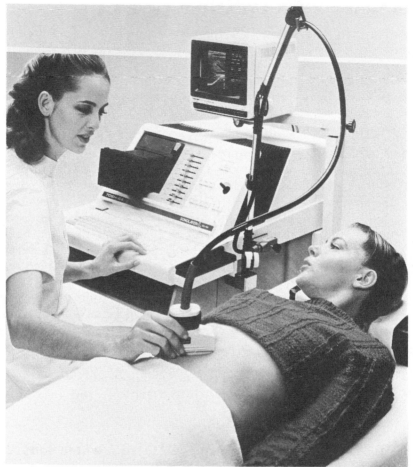

(*Toshiba Corporation*)

Figure 16 A patient having an ultrasound test

showing the density of all the body's structures in the area about which it has rotated. The picture is equivalent to a 'slice' through the body as the beam is narrow (about 1 cm) (Figure 17). The slice shows the different parts of the body clearly as their densities vary. A full examination of the body requires numerous slices so that a three-dimensional picture can be built up. A photographic record of each slice is taken with an instant (polaroid) camera and a more detailed computerized picture can be printed.

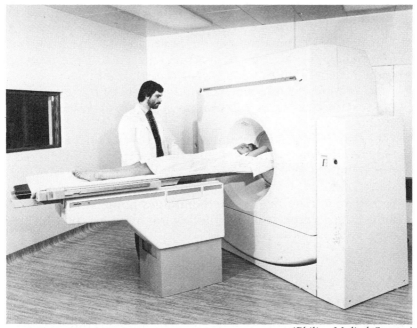

(*Philips Medical Systems*)

Figure 17 A patient about to have a CT scan. The patient will be moved into the centre of the machine as x-rays are taken of the chest and abdomen

- CT scans are not used for routine x-rays as they are expensive and take longer than a normal plain x-ray which is perfectly adequate for most everyday uses. However, when careful examination of small or indistinct structures is required, then the CT scan is the most accurate way of examining the body. It will not replace many of the special x-ray studies previously discussed, but will be used together with other techniques.
- CT scans of the abdomen are usually done after preparation of the bowel. This requires the administration of a laxative for 2 days before the test.
- During the test it may be necessary to get the patient to drink a rather unpleasant tasting liquid as this outlines the stomach and bowel clearly. An injection may also be given to stop the bowel moving, this causes blurred vision for 1–2 hours. During CT scan examinations of the brain, injections of dye may be given

to see if a possible abnormality will absorb the dye and this injection may cause a temporary feeling of heat or discomfort.

- During CT examinations of the brain a close fitting cap may (depending on the type of machine) be put on the head and some patients find this somewhat claustrophobic.
- The duration of a test depends on the extent of the examination but several x-ray slices will be needed so that the test often takes about 1 hour.
- CT scans are painless though sick patients may find them tedious and some patients dislike the dye they may be asked to drink. Injections of contrast dye may be uncomfortable for a short while.
- Most patients are fine to see themselves home after a CT scan unless their vision is blurred following an injection which has been given to slow the bowel.

RADIO ISOTOPE TESTS (isotope imaging or scans)

These tests use injections of very small amounts of radioactive substances which are absorbed by various parts of the body and show up on special photographs taken with a radiation scanner (Figure 18). These tests rely on the radioactive substance, or *isotope*, being specially taken up by the part of the body being examined. Different isotopes are therefore selected for examination of various parts of the body.

Bone scan

A radioactive isotope is used that accumulates in bones that are actively forming new bone. Because of this the picture formed is different from an x-ray as the areas of greatest accumulation of isotope are at sites of bone activity. Increased bone activity (hot areas) may be due to repair of damage (a fracture or arthritis), as well as tumour. Some tumours do not take up the isotope and appear as areas of decreased uptake (cold areas).

- No special preparation is required.
- A painless injection of the isotope is given into a vein in the arm.
- The scan or imaging is done about 2 hours later. The patient lies

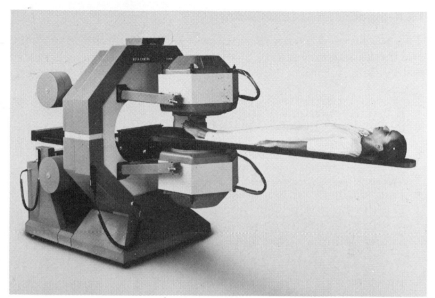

(*Siemens Ltd.*)

Figure 18 A patient about to have an isotope scan. The gamma camera detects the amount of radioactivity in the body and produces a picture

on a firm couch while a radioactive detector or camera produces a picture.
- Patients will be able to drive immediately after the test which should be less than 3 hours from the injection.

Liver scan

The isotope used for this test is taken up by the liver, and areas of the liver that are not working normally will show as a 'hole' as they do not take up the isotope (cold area).

- No special preparation is required.
- A painless injection of isotope is given into an arm vein.
- The scan is done about 20 minutes later and will take about half an hour.
- Patients are able to drive immediately after the test.
- The test takes about 1 hour.

Gall–bladder and biliary scans

This test is used to outline the gall-bladder (containing the bile) and the ducts connecting it to the liver and bowel. The test should not be done for at least one week after a barium meal (page 44).

- No special preparation is necessary.
- A painless injection of isotope is given into a vein in an arm.
- Images or scans of the liver are taken immediately and after several hours. Occasionally a further scan may be done at 24 hours.
- Patients can go home afterwards and are fit to drive.
- The length of time the test takes is variable and depends on how quickly the isotope gets into the gall-bladder. Most tests take less than 4 hours though some patients may need to return for a further scan the next day.

Lung scans

Lung scans can be used to show two things, (a) the blood flow (perfusion) through the lungs, and (b) the flow of air into the lungs (ventilation). Because of this two different isotopes may be used.

- No special preparation is necessary.
- A painless injection of isotope is given into an arm vein (perfusion scan).
- Patients may also be asked to breathe in an isotope (a gas) through an oxygen mask (ventilation).
- Scans of the lungs are taken immediately.
- Patients are able to make their own way home.
- The test should take less than 1 hour.

Thyroid scans

The isotope used for these scans is taken up by the thyroid so that an overactive area shows up as a 'hot spot' and an inactive one as a 'hole' or 'cold area'.

- Patients will be given a list of drugs to avoid before the test. These include iodine, antithyroid drugs, thyroid replacement therapy, and some of the contrast radiological dyes used for special x-rays (page 41). Patients who have not been given a

list, or are in doubt of which drugs or medicines are permissible, should ask the doctor who is to perform the test.
- No other special preparation is needed.
- A painless injection of isotope is given in a vein in an arm.
- Scans of the thyroid are done about 20 minutes later.
- Occasionally patients will be given a dose of isotope by mouth and be asked to return for a scan 24 hours later.
- Patients feel well enough to go home immediately.
- The test should take less than 1 hour.

Kidney (renal) scans

The isotope used is excreted by the kidneys and the function of the kidneys tested.

- No special preparation is required though the test is best done before an IVP (see page 48). If an IVP has been done a gap of 3 days should be left before the scan.
- A painless injection of isotope is given into an arm vein.
- Scanning may begin immediately or may be delayed for 1 hour depending on the information required.
- Patients are able to go home unaccompanied after the test.
- The test should take less than 2 hours.

Other isotope scans

There are other specialized isotope scans which are used occasionally to investigate cancer patients. If you are to have such a scan, discuss the test with your doctor and ask the questions suggested at the end of this section. Nearly all isotope scans are painless and cause little inconvenience.

SPECIAL BIOPSIES

A biopsy, the removal of a small amount of a tissue to examine under the microscope, may be done to make the diagnosis of cancer or to see if a cancer has spread to other tissues. Many tissues can be biopsied and some of the common types of biopsy are discussed below. All biopsies carry a small risk of complications, such as infection or bruising, and it is important to discuss these with the doctor before the test is done.

Lymph node biopsy

Lymph nodes are the glands that respond to infection, they may, for instance, be felt in the neck as painful lumps when a child has tonsillitis. These glands are not confined to the neck but are scattered throughout the body. They are particularly concentrated in the neck, around the collar bones, under the arms, around the major blood vessels in the abdomen, around the heart, and in the groins. In many of these places the lymph nodes are just under the skin so that glands can be felt and if necessary removed surgically — biopsied. The type of surgery and anaesthetic, local or general, will depend on the size and location of the lymph node. Many of these operations are simple and can be done as a day patient. As a cut must be made in the skin, stitches will be put in and will need to be removed about a week later. Occasionally it may be possible to remove a small portion of a lymph node using a needle — a needle biopsy. No anaesthetic or formal operation is then required, though the small size and damaged condition of the tissue may make it more difficult to make a diagnosis when it is examined with a microscope. Patients will need to discuss the need for, methods to be used and side-effects of any biopsy. Following a biopsy the tissue must be prepared before it is examined, and a result will not be available for 24 or more hours. Occasionally sophisticated tests may take several days.

Bone marrow biopsy and aspirate

The *bone marrow* (elements within the bone that form blood) may be sampled to see if it is involved with a cancer or to test the effects of chemotherapy or radiotherapy (discussed later) on its ability to form new blood cells.

- A bone marrow aspirate is done by a small needle which is used to suck some particles from the bone. The test is usually done by locally anaesthetizing or freezing the skin over the breast bone (sternum) and then putting a short needle into the bone. With good local anaesthesia this is not uncomfortable, though there is usually momentary pain when a syringe is used to suck a little of the marrow substance out. The test is done in a few minutes and there should be no side-effects, apart from slight local bruising. The results can be available within a few hours.
- A bone marrow biopsy or trephine is usually done together

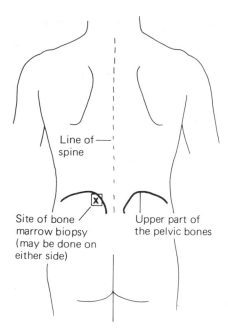

Line of —
spine

Site of bone
marrow biopsy
(may be done on
either side)

Upper part of
the pelvic bones

Figure 19 Diagrammatic representation of the usual site for a bone marrow biopsy

with an aspirate, but because it means removing a small piece of the bone marrow it is not done from the breast bone as this is too thin. Instead it is usually taken from the prominent pelvic bones over the lower back (Figure 19). It may also be done from the pelvic bones forming the border to the front of the abdomen or pelvis. Local anaesthetic is injected to deaden pain though some patients may also require a premedication with a tranquillizer or a pain killer if they are particularly anxious or sensitive to pain. A thin needle is then inserted through the anaesthetized skin into the bone, and is used to remove a small core of bone. This part of the test may be uncomfortable as the local anaesthetic may not deaden *all* the pain from the bone itself. The test should only take a few minutes and many patients do not require extra pain killers. The pain only lasts a short while and there are no long term side-effects of the biopsy.

- Most patients should be able to drive after the test — provided they have not had tranquillizers or pain killers.
- The test may take several days to interpret as the calcium (the bony part) must be removed from the biopsy before it can be examined.

Liver biopsy

Small pieces of tissue may be taken from the liver for examination under a microscope in a variety of conditions; malignant and non-malignant. Liver biopsy requires a short stay in hospital. Before the biopsy is done blood should be examined to ensure that it will clot normally. There may very rarely be some internal bleeding after a biopsy and blood is usually cross-matched in case a transfusion should be required.

- The skin overlying the site of the biopsy (on the right side of the abdomen) is anaesthetized with local anaesthetic. A small cut may then be made so that it is easier to insert the biopsy needle.
- The doctor will explain how he wants the patient to breathe as it is important that the chest and liver are still at the moment of biopsy. Patients are asked to take a deep breath and to then breathe out deeply and hold their breath till the biopsy is done.
- When patient and doctor are happy that this can be done a thin needle is introduced through the anaesthetized skin till it is just over the liver. When the patient has breathed out and the liver is still (it normally moves up and down with each breath) the needle is pushed quickly into and then pulled out of the liver. A syringe is attached to the needle and suction is applied during this movement so that a small piece of liver is sucked into the needle and removed from the liver. There is usually a momentary feeling of pain at this stage of the test which is all over very quickly.
- Patients are then left to rest quietly and their pulse and blood pressure will be recorded regularly for a number of hours. This is to make sure that there has been no internal bleeding from the liver surface. If patients feel pain in the abdomen or over the right shoulder they should call the nurse or doctor. Irritation of the right side of the diaphragm (muscular wall between the

abdomen and chest) often causes pain in the tip of the right shoulder and this may happen without abdominal pain.

- Provided that the patient feels well and the pulse and blood pressure are normal (as in the vast majority) they can go home later, though this will depend on the attitude of the local hospital. Some doctors will do liver biopsies as a day procedure whilst others may ask patients to stay in overnight. The test itself should take less than half an hour.
- There should be little discomfort during the procedure, apart from a jab of pain at the moment of the biopsy. Side-effects are uncommon; if bleeding occurs a blood transfusion may be needed and if it continues an operation may rarely be required. Leakage of bile from the liver is another rare complication that may need to be corrected by operation. It must be stressed that such complications are very unusual, but it is useful to discuss the procedure and its potential complications with the doctor performing the test.
- Some patients often do not feel quite up to normal afterwards so it is best to arrange for someone to accompany them home.
- Tissue from the biopsy is usually ready to be examined within 1–2 days.

Plural biopsy and aspirate

If fluid collects in the space between the lung and chest wall (the pleural space) a biopsy of the lining of the chest wall (the pleura) may be done to determine the cause; usually infection or tumour. In this situation fluid is often drained off the chest (aspirated) regardless of whether a pleural biopsy is done.

- A local anaesthetic is injected into the skin and chest wall between the ribs and often a small cut is made in the skin so that the needle can enter easily. When the chest wall is 'frozen' a short needle is pushed through the small cut into the fluid in the chest. If fluid only is to be removed the needle is attached to a syringe or small suction bottle and the fluid withdrawn. If a pleural biopsy is to be done a small piece of the pleura is cut out in a small notch in the needle. The rest of the fluid may then be removed.
- The moment of the biopsy may be uncomfortable though this should be minimized by a good injection of local anaesthetic.

- If patients experience chest pain, shortness of breath, or a desire to cough, they should tell the doctor. If fluid is removed too quickly the shifting position of the lungs may cause these symptoms which are a sign to stop or abandon the procedure. Most patients feel some of these sensations at the end of the test when the last of the fluid is being removed.
- One complication of the test is a build-up of air in the pleural space between the chest wall and lung (a *pneumothorax*). This may happen if some air gets in by the needle or if the needle scratches the lung surface and causes leakage of air from the lung. Because of this risk a chest x-ray should be performed after the test to check if there has been an air leak. Small amounts of air in the pleural space are not important and can be watched, but large amounts of air will cause collapse of the lung on that side. This complication is unusual, but may mean that a plastic tube must be inserted into the chest to suck out the air. This usually needs to be done for several days to ensure that the lung re-expands.
- The test can often be done as a day procedure, though if the lung collapses from air in the pleural space it will be necessary for the patient to stay in hospital for removal of the air by suction. The test itself takes less than half an hour.
- For those who can go home afterwards it would be best to arrange for someone to collect them.
- Fluid from the chest is sent for examination under a microscope (cytology) as well as the biopsy of the pleura.

Skin biopsy

Biopsy of abnormal areas of the skin are frequently taken to determine whether they are cancerous or not. Very small biopsies may be taken with a special punch, or a larger biopsy may be needed. A punch biopsy only takes a few seconds and is relatively painless. A larger biopsy will require the cutting out of a piece of skin and then stitching the small wound together. Under a good local anaesthetic the procedure should be painless.

- There should be no side-effects.
- The stitches will need to be removed between 5–10 days depending on where the biopsy is.
- Patients should be able to drive after a skin biopsy, provided no sedative has been given.

BLOOD TESTS

The taking of blood (venepuncture) is the commonest type of test in medicine. Blood is taken from a vein in the arm and is used for a wide variety of tests.

- A tight elastic cuff (tourniquet) is put around the upper arm. This slows the blood flow in the veins draining the arm and the veins on the surface stand out because of this.
- When the skin on the arm has been cleaned with a special swab a needle is pushed into the vein and blood sucked into a syringe. Blood is usually taken from the veins in the inside of the elbow though other veins over the back of the arm, hand, or inside of the forearm may be used. Although not normally needed, quite large quantities of blood (100–200 ml) may be taken without *any* side-effects.
- No local anaesthetic is needed and there should be very little discomfort when blood is taken skilfully. Occasionally veins may be difficult and more than one attempt may be necessary. One of the main reasons for failure to get blood is inadequate dilatation (filling) of the veins. If despite a tourniquet the veins do not stand out it may be worth putting the arm into hot water to increase the blood flow. Some patients who have had chemotherapy (drug treatment, Chapter Fourteen) given by injection may have very difficult veins as the drugs often cause clotting and damage to the veins. In such cases blood should only be taken by those used to dealing with these cases.
- After the blood has been taken the needle is removed and a cotton-wool swab is pressed firmly over the needle puncture for a few minutes to prevent bleeding.
- There should be no side-effects apart from a little local bruising.
- Very occasionally patients feel faint when having their blood taken and it is best not to watch the nurse or doctor doing it. The vast majority will be able to leave immediately and can see themselves home.

LARYNGOSCOPY

This is the examination of the voice box (larynx). Although not strictly endoscopy (page 72) it is a similar test as the larynx is not normally available to direct visual examination. A mirror is used for the test.

- A mirror is warmed up (to prevent breath condensing on it).
- The patient is asked to poke his tongue out.
- The tip of the tongue is held by the doctor using some gauze.
- The doctor then puts the mirror (like a dentist's) into the back of the patient's mouth.
- Using a head mirror or light source he looks down the patient's throat at the larynx.

The test is only mildly uncomfortable if done expertly and takes a few minutes.

CERVICAL SMEAR (PAP SMEAR)

As there are rarely early signs or symptoms of *cervical cancer* (cancer of the cervix or neck of the womb, page 160) it has become normal to examine the surface of the cervix when a pelvic examination is done.

- During the pelvic examination the walls of the vagina are held apart with an instrument called a speculum, so that the cervix can be seen. A wooden spatula is then scraped over the surface of the cervix and the cells on the spatula are then smeared on a glass slide. After the cells have been stained they are examined under a microscope to check if there are any early signs of cancer.
- The examination should be only slightly uncomfortable.
- No special preparation is required and patients have no side-effects after the test.
- Results of the test are usually ready in a day or so. It should be done periodically when screening for cervical cancer.

DIRECT VISUAL EXAMINATIONS INSIDE THE BODY (endoscopy)

Sigmoidoscopy

A sigmoidoscopy is an examination of the rectum and last part of the large bowel (Figure 20). A lubricated stainless steel tube is passed gently into the back passage (rectum). This has a light inside so that the operator can see into the rectum. It is also connected to a hand-operated bulb which pumps air at low

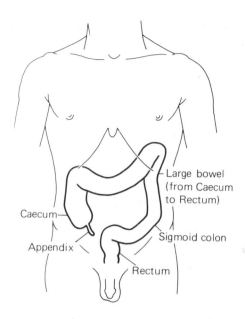

Figure 20 Diagrammatic representation of the course of the large bowel

pressure into the rectum and expands the large bowel. As the bowel is expanded so the sigmoidoscope (the tube in the rectum) can be pushed further into the large bowel. Using this instrument it is possible to examine up to 18 cm of the last part of the large bowel. As most cancers develop in this area, it is an important examination. It is possible, using a wire snare or swab, to remove small polyps from the bowel for microscopic examination.

- Apart from mild discomfort the test is painless.
- No preparation is required though the test cannot be done if the rectum is loaded with faeces.
- There are no side-effects and patients are able to leave immediately and to drive.

Colonoscopy

This is a method of looking into the large bowel using an instrument called a colonoscope. A sigmoidoscope is a straight metal tube and it can only be used to examine the last part of the large bowel (rectum and sigmoid colon). A colonoscope is made from optical fibres which can be bent and the instrument can be guided around curves so that the whole of the large bowel (Figure 20) can be examined. The colonoscope transmits a bright light and allows the doctor to look into the bowel. As light follows the curve of the fibres it is possible to see round corners.

- Preparation of the bowel is necessary and patients will be given instructions to take laxatives for two days before the test. An enema may be used prior to the test to ensure that the bowel is empty.
- The test is usually done as an out-patient, though many hospitals admit patients to a day ward.
- A sedative may be given prior to the test.
- The lubricated colonoscope is then passed into the rectum whilst the patient lies curled up on their side.
- The instrument is gradually advanced into the large bowel and the inside of the bowel examined on the way and photographs can be taken if required.
- It is usually possible to examine the whole of the large bowel and to biopsy (page 65) any polyps on the way. A snare is used to remove the polyp, often with a hook being used to hold it. This should not be unduly uncomfortable.
- The test is finished when the colonoscopy is removed. There may be some discomfort with the investigation, but this should not be severe.
- Patients can leave immediately after the test but should arrange for a taxi or someone to collect them and should not drive after a sedative.

Gastroscopy

This is the use of a flexible instrument to look into the gullet (oesophagus), stomach, and upper small bowel (duodenum) (see Figure 21). The gastroscope is made from optical fibres which can be bent. The doctor performing the investigation is able to guide the gastroscope so that he can look around the stomach. There are two types of gastroscope, (a) forward viewing, and (b) side viewing. Either may be used though each is better at particular types of examination. As far as the patient is concerned there is no difference between the way the two types are used.

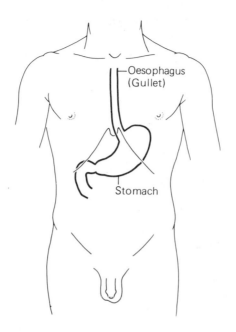

Figure 21 Diagrammatic representation of the upper gastrointestinal tract

- You will be asked not to eat or drink from the night before the test. This is to ensure that there is no food in the stomach.
- The test is usually done as an out-patient, though many hospitals admit their patients to a day ward.
- A sedative is given before the test and this is often an injection into a vein which will make the patient sleepy, reduces discomfort, and means that they often remember little of the actual test. Local anaesthetic is also sprayed into the back of the throat to reduce discomfort and a tendency to gag.
- When preparations are complete the lubricated end of the gastroscope is guided into the patient's mouth and throat so that it is swallowed into the gullet or oesophagus. The gullet is examined visually as the instrument is passed into the stomach. Photographs may be taken at any part of the test.
- As the gastroscope is passed further it comes into the stomach. The doctor can then manoeuvre the tip of the instrument to examine all parts of the stomach.

- The tip can also be guided into the last part of the stomach as it becomes the duodenum. This area between the duodenum and stomach is a common site of ulcers. The gastroscope is passed through into the duodenum and the entrance of the bile duct and duct from the pancreas can be examined. In addition to examining and photographing any suspicious areas, biopsies (page 65) may be taken. This should not cause any discomfort.
- When the test is completed the gastroscope is taken out.
- Because a strong sedative has been used patients will need to rest and recover from the test.
- Patients should not drive after the test as they have had a sedative injection.
- The test will take about 1 hour but time for recovery from the sedative is needed so that patients should expect to be at the hospital for most of the day.

ERCP (examination of the ducts to the gall-bladder and pancreas)

ERCP (standing for, in medical language, endoscopic retrograde cholangiopancreatography) is a test using a gastroscope (see above) to examine and then inject x-ray contrast dye into the ducts from the gall-bladder and pancreas, as they enter the duodenum (Figure 22).

- A gastroscopy is carried out. This requires the same preparation as described in the previous section.
- When the gastroscope is in the duodenum the tiny entrance to the ducts is identified. They usually enter the bowel through a small raised area known as the ampulla of Vater. A fine plastic tube (catheter) is passed down the gastroscope and into the opening of the duct. The doctor can select either the bile duct or the pancreatic duct. The test is difficult and requires a skilled gastroscopist. When the catheter is in the duct a small amount of x-ray dye is injected and a series of x-rays taken.
- The test itself may take about 1 hour.
- Recovery time is required after the sedative.
- Patients should *not* attempt to drive home and will need to be collected.
- The test is usually done as an out-patient though admission to a day ward is common.

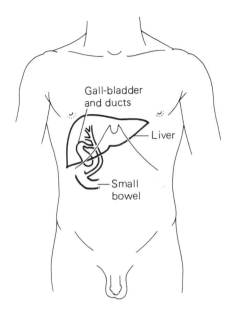

Figure 22 Diagrammatic representation of the duct from the gall–bladder to the small bowel; the pancreatic duct joins the bowel in the same place and both may be examined during the ERCP

Bronchoscopy

Bronchoscopy is a test where a doctor looks directly into the main air-ways into the lung (bronchi) (Figure 23). In the past rigid metal bronchoscopes were used but the introduction of flexible fibre-optic bronchoscopes has made the test much easier. The optical fibres in these new bronchoscopes can be bent and transmit light into the chest and allow the doctor to see into the main air-ways.

- The test can be done as an out-patient though patients may be admitted to hospital.
- Sedation is usually given before the test.
- The back of the throat is sprayed with a local anaesthetic to reduce discomfort and the tendency to gagging.
- The flexible bronchoscope is usually thin and is passed into the back of the throat through a nostril.
- Photographs can be taken during the examination and pieces of tumour (biopsies) taken for examination.

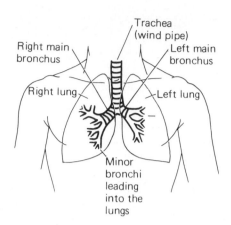

Figure 23 Diagrammatic representation of the main airways leading into the lungs. These can be examined through a bronchoscope

QUESTIONS TO ASK ABOUT INVESTIGATIONS

If further information on the tests described or other more specialized investigations not discussed is required, these questions may be useful.

(1) Why is the test necessary?
(2) How is the test done?
(3) Is any preparation needed?
(4) Is the test uncomfortable or unpleasant?
(5) Are there any immediate side-effects?
(6) How long does the test take?
(7) Are there any long term side-effects?
(8) Will I need to be admitted to hospital for the test?
(9) If not, can I go home on my own and am I safe to drive?

CHAPTER TWELVE

Surgery for cancer

Surgery was the first effective treatment of cancer and is still the usual treatment for many localized tumours. During this century more complicated surgery has become routine, not only because of improved surgical techniques, but perhaps more importantly better anaesthetic and post-operative care.

Surgery is important because it cures more patients of cancer than radiotherapy and drug therapy together. This chapter examines the various roles of surgery in the treatment of cancer.

DIAGNOSIS

Before the diagnosis of cancer can be made a biopsy *must* be taken. A biopsy (page 65) is the surgical removal of a sample of tissue, such as a lymph node, for examination under a microscope. A biopsy is taken when there is a suspicious lump but will often show that there is no cancer and may occasionally be done when cancer is not suspected. Biopsies are usually performed by surgeons though some of the tests may be done by other doctors. They are frequently done under local anaesthetic or as a day procedure.

There are several ways to obtain a sample of tissue. The method used depends on the site of the possible cancer and the size of the biopsy needed. Common types of biopsy are listed below and are described more fully in the section on investigations.

- Excision biopsy. This is the surgical removal of the whole tumour. This is frequently done for small tumours of the breast and skin cancers; If a lump can be removed in one piece this is ideal.
- Incisional biopsy. Only part of the lump is removed during this procedure. It is usually done when the lump is too large to be removed easily.
- Needle biopsy. A needle is inserted into a lump and part of the tissue or fluid within the tumour is cut or sucked out.

● Endoscopic biopsy. When a tube is passed into the body to see areas that are not normally visible the technique is known as endoscopy (page 72). Biopsies of small pieces of tissue may be taken using the tube or endoscope. The common types of tests are:

(a) Gastroscopy and oesophagoscopy, examination of the gullet, stomach, and first part of bowel (page 74).
(b) Sigmoidoscopy, examination of rectum and last part of bowel (page 72).
(c) Colonoscopy, examination of the large bowel (page 73).
(d) Bronchoscopy, examination of the air passages into the lungs (page 77).
(e) Cystoscopy, examination of the urinary bladder.
(f) Laryngoscopy, examination of the throat and voice box.
(g) Colposcopy, examination of the cervix (neck of the womb) and vaginal examination.

STAGING (see Chapters Ten and Eleven)

Although most staging is done by special x-rays and other tests surgeons are asked to help to stage certain types of tumour. In Hodgkin's disease (page 202) examination and removal of the spleen and lymph nodes within the abdomen may be done when the disease is found to be at an early stage by routine tests. This operation is called a staging laparotomy. Such operations for staging are only done in a few special cancers and most surgical staging procedures consist of needle biopsies or certain types of endoscopy. Staging is often crucial for the choice of treatment and surgical examination and removal of tissue may be the most accurate way of finding how much a cancer has spread.

CURATIVE SURGERY FOR LOCALIZED CANCER

If a tumour has not spread to distant parts of the body then it is potentially curable with surgery or radiotherapy. It is crucial that all the cancerous tissue is removed, or the tumour will recur.

It is therefore essential that all tumour that can be seen together with a wide margin of normal tissue is removed. This may result in an operation that is disfiguring — such as a mastectomy for breast cancer or removal of a tumour of the head or neck.

Although the surgery may seem mutilating the choice lies between disfigurement or a spreading tumour which could end in death.

Surgeons will often attempt to remove nearby lymph nodes. If these are taken with the original tumour in one piece the operation is called *en bloc* resection. More distant draining lymph nodes may also be removed in the case of certain tumours. This is because the surgeon knows that the risk of spread is high, even though they may not appear abnormal.

SURGERY TO CONTROL SYMPTOMS

Operations designed to control or prevent symptoms but not to cure are called 'palliative'. No attempt is made to remove all the tumour; the operation is designed to deal with specific problems. If, for instance, the bowel is obstructed by a tumour that cannot be removed, the surgeon can by-pass the obstruction so that pain caused by the obstruction is relieved. The pain and effects of the operation must be balanced against the possible gains and the patient's life expectancy. Careful thought is required before palliative surgery, but its use can be of great benefit to patients and can prolong life.

SURGERY TO PREVENT CANCER

The removal of growths that may if left turn into cancers is commonly forgotten, but is important in certain tumours. Perhaps the commonest operation is the removal of polyps from the colon. Rarely, drastic operations such as removal of the colon for familial polyposis (page 13) or chronic ulcerative colitis (page 15) are needed when the risk of cancer is very high.

EFFECTS OF SURGERY

(1) Following surgery there is inevitably some pain. The amount of pain depends very much upon the operation but the use of pain killers should control most pain.
(2) Infection at the site of operation is a potential risk but with good surgical technique is usually avoided.
(3) After major operations clots may form in veins in the legs and pelvis. Occasionally these may break off and end up in

the lungs (a pulmonary embolus; patients are encouraged to move their legs after an operation to try to avoid this).

(4) Chest infections are not uncommon after a general anaesthetic and physiotherapy is given to the chest before and after a major operation.

The likelihood of side-effects (or even death in very few patients) varies according to the operation and patients need to discuss all this fully before surgery. The questions below may be useful in such a discussion.

● Questions to ask before an operation

(1) General questions

Why is this operation being chosen, and what exactly will be done?
Are there any other ways of dealing with the problem besides surgery?
What is the usual stay in hospital and how long before I am really fit?
How much pain will there be?
What about cigarettes? are they dangerous, should I give them up before coming into hospital?
Where will the scar be, will it be obvious?
Will there be any other treatment afterwards?

(2) Biopsy

How will the biopsy be done?
Will an anaesthetic be necessary?
If the biopsy shows cancer, will the surgeon carry on to a full operation at the same time?
Is it necessary to stay in hospital overnight after the biopsy?
Should I arrange transport or can I see myself home?
Are there any side-effects?

(3) Curative surgery

Why is the operation being done?
Are there any other alternatives to an operation?

Is any special preparation necessary?
How long will I have to stay afterwards?
Is the operation uncomfortable and are there any possible side-effects?
Does anyone ever die from the operation?
Where will the scar be and is it disfiguring?
Is any special appliance needed afterwards, such as a colostomy?
Will any further operation be needed?
Is any other treatment planned?

The surgeon may not be able to give a definite answer to all of these questions before an operation, as the exact procedure will depend on the stage of the cancer found at the operation, but should be able to give an idea of what to expect.

(4) Palliative surgery (to prevent symptoms)

How will the operation help or prevent symptoms?
How much pain is caused by the operation?
Will the operation have other unwanted effects?
Does anyone ever die from the operation?
How long will I be in hospital?
Are there other ways of treating or preventing the symptoms?

CHAPTER THIRTEEN

Radiotherapy for cancer

Radiotherapy (also called radiation therapy, deep x-ray therapy, cobalt treatment, or irradiation) is the use of high energy rays to kill cancer cells. Most radiotherapy is given by a machine some distance away from the patient (external therapy) though small amounts of radioactive material (implants) may be placed inside the body for a few days during internal therapy.

Radiation damages the ability of cells to divide and multiply; this affects both normal and cancer cells and all cells are sensitive to irradiation if a high enough dose is given. The dose of radiotherapy that can be given safely depends on the effect of the irradiation on the normal tissues. A dose that does not cause severe side-effects is used and this will often kill cancer cells within a tumour and reduce its size or destroy it completely. Because many tumours are more easily damaged by radiation than normal tissues a useful response to the treatment results.

Radiotherapy can be used in a variety of ways. In some cancers it may totally destroy the tumour and will cure the patients. In other situations where a tumour is too large to be removed surgically radiotherapy is sometimes used to shrink the cancer so that it can be surgically taken away. It may also be used together with drug treatment (chemotherapy) to get the best response in certain cancers and is also very useful in reducing a wide variety of symptoms, including pain.

In recent times there have been important improvements in the use of radiotherapy. These changes are a result of increasing information on the dose of radiotherapy that normal tissues can withstand. Modern machines used to give the treatment can now deliver more radiation to a cancer whilst giving a smaller dose to the surrounding normal tissues and skin. The other major improvement in radiotherapy has come from a greater under-standing of the normal behaviour of cancers by doctors using radiotherapy (radiotherapists or radiation therapists).

HOW IS RADIOTHERAPY GIVEN?

- The first visit to a radiotherapy department usually does not involve treatment. A radiotherapist first will talk about the treatment and make an examination prior to starting radiotherapy. There may well be further x-rays or other tests to define the site of the cancer and treatment is then 'planned'. During the treatment planning the area (field or portal) to be treated is marked out on the skin. A purple dye (which must not be washed off) may be used or some small tattoos (dots, only) are used to outline the corners of the field. After this has been done the radiotherapist will work with a radiation physicist to calculate the dose of radiation needed. This will depend on the type of cancer, the site involved, and the person's body shape. The word most commonly used to describe the dose is called rads (radiation absorbed dose) and it refers to the amount of radiation absorbed by the tissue.

- Treatment usually consists of a series of individual treatments which are called fractions. The number of fractions needed will again depend on several factors. Treatment may be almost daily (Monday–Friday) for an average of about 3–4 weeks. Those about to receive radiotherapy should ask how often the treatment is given and how long it is planned to continue the treatment (remembering that the plan may need to be changed). The treatment is split into fractions in order to protect the normal tissues; it is more effective to give small doses of radiotherapy each day than to give one large dose.

- What are the machines like? Although there are different types of radiotherapy machine, most people's immediate reaction is of 'how enormous and complex they are' (Figure 24). Not only are they big but the machine or table that the patient lies on may move up or down or rotate, often with a humming noise. The whole complicated machine and its array of controls is designed to give a carefully designed dose of radiotherapy with safety. It is normal for anyone to feel frightened by the machinery but one rapidly becomes used to it.

- The treatment is given by a radiographer specially trained in giving radiotherapy. Using the tattoos or painted markers they will position the person on the table for treatment. Parts of the body may be protected by lead blocks placed above or on the body. For certain tumours a plastic shield may be used to

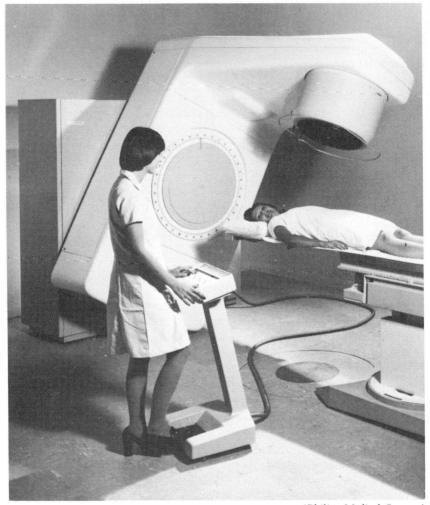

(*Philips Medical Systems*)

Figure 24 Modern radiotherapy machine (a linear accelerator)

reduce any movement during treatment. This is particularly common during radiation therapy to the head where it is important to lie quite still during treatment to make sure the area treated is exactly the same each time. Plastic shields or moulds are often specially made for individual patients and special measurements may be taken before treatment can start.

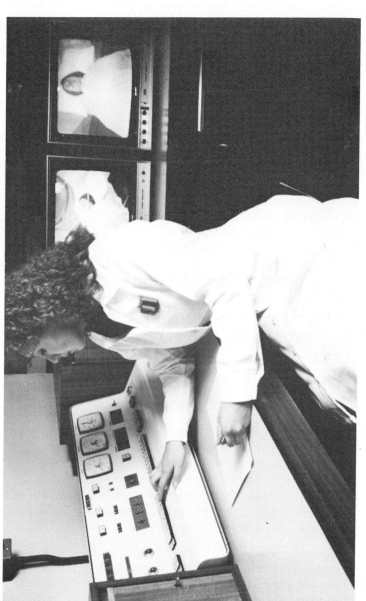

(Philips Medical Systems)

Figure 25 A radiographer controlling radiotherapy treatment. The patient can be seen on a television screen behind the radiographer and she can talk to him through an intercom

- The radiographer will not stay in the room during the treatment. She will control the treatment from another room and will be able to see the patient on a TV screen or through a thick window and can talk to them through a loudspeaker system (Figure 25). Patients are watched throughout the treatment, which usually only takes a few minutes.
- Various types of equipment may be used according to the cancer. Orthovoltage radiotherapy machines (of relatively low energy) were one of the first type of equipment used to treat cancer. Their main disadvantages are an inability to penetrate skin well and difficulty in focusing the beam so that surrounding normal tissue is treated as well. Because, in the past, doctors tried to use it to give high doses to internal tumours, it often caused skin burns which gave radiotherapy a bad name. It is now only used in special circumstances and does not cause severe burns as the doses are lower. Cobalt and linear accelerators are more modern machines that give high doses to the tumour and less to the skin. They can be focused and the dose to surrounding tissues is low. Most cancers are now treated on one or other of these machines. Other special machines use different types of radiation but are experimental at present.

No one is radioactive from treatment and they should not feel a risk to other people.

SIDE-EFFECTS OF RADIOTHERAPY

As radiation effects both normal and cancer cells it is not surprising that it causes side-effects. Side-effects do not happen to all patients, and their severity varies from person to person. The type and degree of side-effects depends on the part of the body being treated, the dose of radiotherapy, the way it is split up into fractions, and any other drug treatment (especially anticancer drugs) that may be given at the same time.

- The most common side-effect of radiation is tiredness. This may build up during treatment but will improve in the first few weeks after stopping treatment. Along with tiredness many patients lose their appetite and some feel sick. Advice on eating during therapy is given on page 340.

- Many patients notice slight reddening of the skin, like sunburn, and tanning of the treated skin is common at the end of the radiotherapy. This is expected and will clear up. If, as occasionally happens, the skin starts to break down and weep patients should tell their radiotherapist or radiographer. It is important to take care of the skin being treated and soaps, perfumes, cosmetics, hot-water bottles, and UV or heat lamps should not be used at all on the area being treated. Ointments should not be put on the area without asking the radiotherapist's advice and the area should be protected from sunlight or extreme cold. Patients who need to shave should use an electric razor if the skin of the face is being treated.

- Diarrhoea. When the abdomen is being treated, diarrhoea may be a problem. Patients with diarrhoea should tell their radiotherapist who may prescribe specific treatment. The following suggestions may be helpful for controlling the symptoms. A clear liquid diet (page 34) can be tried to see if this will allow the diarrhoea to settle. Avoid foods that may cause cramping — these include spirits, spicy foods, coffee, cabbage, cauliflower, broccoli, and baked beans. If a liquid diet does not get rid of the diarrhoea small amounts of food should be eaten frequently and plenty of fluids drunk. Milk products are usually not helpful and should be avoided. As the diarrhoea improves, soft low fibre foods (page 343) should be added into the diet.

- Radiotherapy to the head and neck may cause particular side-effects. A sore throat on swallowing or eating can be troublesome. If this is the case, the patient's diet should be changed to a soft diet of well cooked foods. All solids should be cut up into small bites and moistened with gravy; spicy foods and spirits should be avoided. If necessary, the diet should be supplemented with liquid high calorie and protein drinks such as Complan (page 300). Radiotherapists may prescribe a liquid local anaesthetic (page 30) that should be drunk before eating so that pain on swallowing is reduced.

- If the radiotherapy area includes the mouth, patients should take special care of their teeth. Patients with bad teeth should preferably see their dentist before treatment and tell him that they are going to receive radiotherapy. Teeth should be cleaned regularly (up to 4 times a day) with a soft round bristle brush and a smooth fluoride toothpaste used. After cleaning their teeth patients can rinse out their mouth with a solution of salt and baking soda (1 teaspoon of each to 1 quart of warm water); most commercial mouth washes should be avoided as they contain alcohol.

- Radiation to the jaws will also affect the salivary glands so that they produce less saliva. Patients who develop a sore mouth, should drink plenty of fluids and rinse their mouth out frequently to get rid of food debris which would normally be swallowed with saliva. Some patients find it useful to suck ice cubes. If the problem is chronic fluoride mouth washes or artificial saliva can be used.

- A change in taste is common during radiotherapy to the mouth. This may be a simple loss of taste or may make certain foods unpleasant. Patients need to experiment with foods to see which taste best and try to prepare foods that look or smell good even if they cannot taste them.

- If the radiotherapy includes the scalp *temporary* hair loss occurs. This is very upsetting, and is difficult to adjust to, but the hair will start to grow back after treatment. Many patients have wigs whilst they have lost their hair (they are supplied by the National Health Service in Britain) and others wear hats or scarves.

- Radiation to the testes or ovaries will usually result in loss of fertility. The testes are specially sensitive to radiotherapy.

Other side-effects of radiotherapy are less common and depend on the area being treated and it is important that patients discuss possible side-effects with their radiotherapist before treatment.

Many patients feel 'down' or depressed during treatment; this is probably a result of several factors. Worry about the diagnosis of cancer, about the type of treatment they are having, together with a sudden change in their daily routine and the side-effects of the treatment all cause depression. This is normal, but it is useful for patients to discuss their feelings with relatives and friends as well as the doctors and nurses looking after them.

With all radiation there is a *small* long term risk that the treatment itself may cause a second cancer. Such tumours are uncommon and usually do not occur for a number of years (up to 20 years).

QUESTIONS TO ASK ABOUT THE SIDE-EFFECTS OF RADIOTHERAPY

(1) Will I feel tired?
(2) Will I feel sick?
(3) Are there any specific side-effects caused by the particular type of radiotherapy I am receiving?
(4) How long will the side-effects last?
(5) Are any special precautions required?
(6) Are there any long term effects of the treatment?
(7) Will the radiotherapy affect my fertility?

RADIATION IMPLANT THERAPY

When certain tumours are being treated a small container of radioactive material may be placed (implanted) into a patient's body. The way that the radioactive material is implanted depends on the area to be treated, and the radiotherapist should discuss the details with the patient.

Patients are usually admitted to hospital for this procedure and an anaesthetic may be necessary. The stay in hospital varies but is often less than one week. Patients are usually in a single room to protect others from the radiation of the implant, and visiting may be restricted and patients be asked to stay in bed so as not to displace the implant.

Side-effects depend on where the implant is and patients should ask their doctor about this. The radioactive implant will be removed before the patient goes home and is then no longer a risk to other people.

GENERAL QUESTIONS ABOUT RADIOTHERAPY

Patients should discuss their treatment fully with their doctor before starting. It is sometimes useful to write the questions down before seeing a doctor and to make a note of answers.

(1) Why do I need radiotherapy?
(2) Are there alternative treatments?
(3) Which part of me will be treated with the radiation?
(4) How long will the treatment take?
(5) How often will the treatment be given?

(6) How long does each treatment take?
(7) Can I drive, or do I need transport home?
(8) What are the general or particular side-effects? (Page 88).
(9) Should I take any special precautions during treatment?

Patients having any difficulties during treatment should tell their doctor.

CHAPTER FOURTEEN

Drug treatment (chemotherapy) of cancer

Chemotherapy (a shortened version of chemical therapy) means the use of drugs and hormones to treat disease. Although the word can be applied to other drug treatments, it is commonly used to mean the drug treatment of cancer.

Only thirty years ago there were no useful drugs for the treatment of cancer. The speciality of chemotherapy or medical oncology (the medical or drug treatment of tumours) is therefore very new. From the first discovery of anticancer drugs in the late 1940s there has been a rapid development of drug therapy, and this continues.

One of the major drawbacks of surgery and radiotherapy is that they only treat locally — that is, only the tissue removed or irradiated is treated. Chemotherapy treats the whole body and cancer which has spread and is beyond local treatment is affected. Drug treatment is, however, often given in combination with surgery or radiotherapy.

HOW DO THE DRUGS WORK?

It is beyond the scope of this book to describe in detail the way each type of drug works. There are over thirty commonly used anticancer drugs, and each has different ways of affecting cells though they often fall into broad groups or classes of drugs acting similarly. A list of the common classes of drugs, their uses and common side-effects are shown in Appendix A.

- All cancer drugs basically work by poisoning cells. They damage or kill cells so that they are unable to divide and multiply and unfortunately they harm both normal and cancer cells. Despite major efforts we have failed to develop drugs which only attack cancerous cells and successful treatment depends on damaging tumour cells more than normal cells.

93

- High doses damage more cells. Medical oncologists frequently use high doses of drugs to kill as many tumour cells as possible; this will, of course, cause side-effects. If high-dose treatment can cure or greatly prolong life then most doctors and patients feel that it is worthwhile; but for tumours that do not respond well to chemotherapy, toxic treatment should be avoided as it may do more harm than good.
- Most anticancer drugs kill or damage cells best when the cells are dividing. The normal cells in the body that divide rapidly are in the bone marrow (making new blood), in the bowel (making new lining cells), in the hair follicles, in the testis (making sperm), and in the skin. Because of this the common side-effects (page 99) of chemotherapy are mainly in these parts of the body. Many cancers have cells that are dividing rapidly, though this alone does not explain the effectiveness of anti-cancer drugs and, unfortunately, there are also cells within tumours that are not dividing. Some drugs will attack these cells and scientists are looking for more drugs like these.
- The larger a cancer is the slower its cells are dividing. Since drugs are most effective against rapidly dividing cells it is only to be expected that anticancer drugs are most useful in small tumours. Because the blood supply of large tumours is poor, the ability of drugs to get into a big tumour is also affected. These two factors mean that chemotherapy is best given when tumours have not grown to a large size though it does not mean that drugs cannot be effective in a large responsive tumour, only that the chances are reduced.
- During the early years of chemotherapy a single drug was commonly used by itself. Despite some effect, tumours usually grew back and drugs are now usually used together in a combination. It is thought that single drugs fail because the cancer develops a way of overcoming their effects. This is less likely if several drugs, working in different ways, are used together. As well as choosing drugs that act differently, doctors try to put together drugs that have different side-effects so that high doses of all the drugs can be given.
- So that big doses of the drugs can be used it is usual to allow several weeks between each treatment. Chemotherapy is, therefore, often given at 3–4 weekly intervals. Some treatments, especially those taken by mouth, may be given continuously.

WHEN SHOULD CHEMOTHERAPY BE USED?

The drugs used in cancer chemotherapy cause more side-effects than probably any other medicines. For this reason it is very important that they are only used when they will benefit the patient.

If the treatment is likely to be curative then chemotherapy that causes side-effects is usually acceptable both to the patient and doctor. It is more difficult to decide if chemotherapy is helpful when the chance of a good response is small or if the aim of the treatment is purely to relieve symptoms (palliative treatment). When doctors and patients consider drug treatment of cancer they must always weigh the potential advantages of the treatment against the side-effects. Such a balance is frequently complex, and patients should discuss the need for treatment, its aims and disadvantages. The usefulness of chemotherapy is changing rapidly and patients *must* discuss their own particular treatment with their doctor.

● Cancers that can be cured with chemotherapy

There is a small but growing list of cancers that can be cured with drugs used alone or together with other treatments. These include acute lymphatic leukaemia in children, Wilm's tumour in children (a kidney cancer), rhabdomyosarcoma in children (a tumour of muscle), osteogenic sarcoma in children (a tumour of bones), lymphomas in children (cancer of lymph glands), Hodgkin's disease (a cancer of lymph glands), testicular cancer, chorio-carcinoma in women (cancer of the tissue of the placenta after child birth), lymphomas in adults (cancer of the lymph glands).

Most of the cancers on this list are relatively uncommon. The treatment of several includes hospital admission and a lot of drug side-effects but most patients will accept these disadvantages for a chance of cure.

● Chemotherapy that reduces symptoms or prolongs life (palliation)

Many advanced tumours cannot, yet, be cured by chemotherapy. Relief of symptoms and prolongation of life is, however, possible in some of these cancers. If palliative chemotherapy is planned then there must be a clear goal; the trade-off in terms of toxic side-effects must be worthwhile. Toxicity is discussed more fully later in this chapter, but if palliative treatment is planned a thorough discussion of side-effects is essential. Chemotherapy may be of some benefit in the following cancers; almost all childhood cancers if not curable will respond to drugs, cancer of the breast, ovary, oat cell (small cell) cancer of the lung, acute leukaemia in adults, multiple myeloma, cancer of the prostate, cancer of the thyroid, some adult sarcomas, and cancer of the pancreas.

Cancers that do not respond to chemotherapy

Chemotherapy is not very effective in some of the common cancers. This is not to say that they never respond; only that useful antitumour effects are infrequent. When the benefits of chemotherapy are uncertain the side-effects of treatment must be considered with great care. If there is no successful treatment then only treatment which has few side-effects should be considered, unless patients are willing or anxious to be treated with new experimental drugs (see Chapter Twenty).

The following cancers often respond poorly to chemotherapy: cancers of the colon and rectum, oesophagus, stomach, mouth, bladder, cervix, brain, non-small cell lung cancer (page 194), and malignant melanoma. Occasionally patients do benefit from treatment; those most likely to respond are patients who feel well before treatment and who have relatively small tumours. Large tumours in very sick patients almost never respond usefully to chemotherapy and drug treatment is best avoided in such patients. The tumours on these lists are gradually changing and with time more tumours will become treatable and eventually curable.

HOW IS CHEMOTHERAPY GIVEN?

Anticancer chemotherapy is usually given in one of three ways.

  (a) By mouth, some drugs are given as tablets or capsules.
  (b) Intramuscularly, a *few* drugs are given by injection into a muscle or under the skin.
  (c) Intravenously, many of the drugs are given by an injection into a vein on the forearm. A small needle is put through the skin into a vein and the drug solution injected slowly

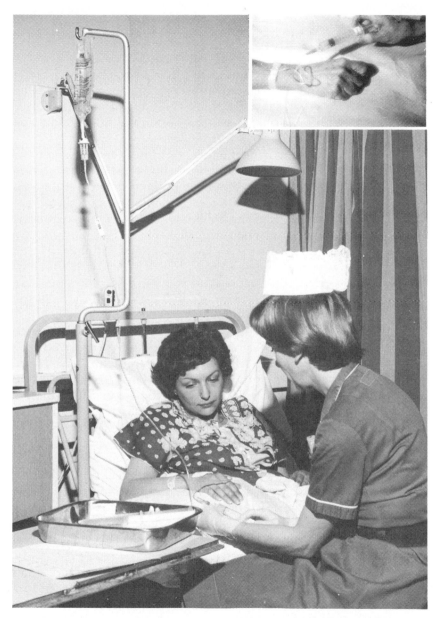

Figure 26 A patient being given a chemotherapy drug into a vein. An intravenous infusion (drip) is set up and the drug is injected into the fluid running into a vein on the arm. The inset photograph shows a small needle, known as a butterfly, being used for an injection into a vein on the forearm

(Figure 26). This should be relatively painless though it can become difficult to find good veins in patients who have had a lot of chemotherapy.

- For some drugs the intravenous needle is connected to a bottle containing a salt solution (an infusion) and the drug injected into the fluid running into the vein. Occasionally the drug may be mixed with the solution in the bottle and allowed to run slowly into the vein over a longer period.
- Many patients ask if chemotherapy is painful. On the whole the answer is no. Occasionally the intravenous injection of certain drugs may cause a burning sensation in the vein and a mild pain may last for some hours after treatment. Putting the intravenous needle into a vein should be quite easy in most patients, but as treatment progresses the veins may be damaged by repeated tests and treatment so that it becomes difficult to get a needle in the vein. Patients should tell the doctor or nurse of any pain experienced when a drug is being injected. This may be a sign to stop the injection as some drugs will damage the skin if they leak from the vein.
- If it becomes difficult to give treatment because of damaged veins, then a long plastic line or catheter may be placed in a larger vein. Recent use of special long catheters has made treatment easier for some patients having very intensive treatment. The major advantage of these special catheters (known as Hickman lines) is that they can be left in place throughout the treatment. All drugs, transfusions, etc. can be given through this line and blood can be withdrawn for tests. Disadvantages are the small operation required to put the line in and the scrupulous care required to prevent infection or clotting in the catheter. Nevertheless, it may be of benefit to patients receiving intensive treatment or those who have very poor veins in their arms. Not all centres use these lines, but they are being more commonly used when a patient is about to start a period of intensive treatment.
- Slow infusions of drugs are given to some patients and small portable pumps are becoming available. A needle is placed in a vein as usual and this is connected by a short plastic line to a pump containing the drug and this injects the drug slowly at the required rate. This is a recent development that is becoming more commonly used in the United States.

WHAT ARE THE SIDE-EFFECTS OF CHEMOTHERAPY?

Side-effects vary from drug to drug and person to person. Not everyone will have side-effects and it is important that a doctor explains the sort of toxicity that they can expect. This may be minimal or quite severe, depending on the drugs given. However, even if patients are told that the side-effects may be severe some may be lucky and get away with little inconvenience. The more common side-effects are discussed in this section; remember this is a list, and patients must discuss the *specific* effects of the therapy they will receive. Appendix A includes the common side-effects of the major anticancer drugs. It is also important to see if you will be able to work or carry on as normal during treatment. Experience will allow the doctor to give a fairly accurate assessment of what to expect, but patients will have a better idea after the first treatment as the pattern of side-effects is usually similar with each course of treatment.

Tiredness and malaise.

Occurs with many chemotherapy treatments. Patients feel tired and unwell, 'one degree under' is a common description. This may gradually get worse during the treatment, though it commonly improves between each course or cycle of treatment.

Decreased appetite, nausea, and vomiting.

One of the most troublesome side-effects of some anticancer drugs is nausea and vomiting. Patients will be given treatment (tablets, suppositories, or possibly injections) to help control the nausea. In those patients who develop this side-effect it usually starts within a few hours of treatment and is over by 12 hours, though occasionally patients may be nauseated for several days. The drugs which most frequently cause nausea and vomiting (see Appendix A) are cis platin, nitrogen mustard, adriamycin, cyclophosphamide, CCNU, BCNU, actinomycin D, dauno-mycin, and DTIC. The severity of the nausea varies markedly between patients but if vomiting is severe patients may need to be hospitalized to prevent dehydration and to make sure that the best antisickness treatment is given.

Patients may be able to help minimize the side-effect at home by:

(1) Eating small frequent meals for a day or so after treatment.
(2) Not drinking liquids with meals to avoid filling the stomach. Drinking frequent small amounts of clear fluids between meals.
(3) Avoiding spicy, fried, or fatty foods.
(4) Eating slowly and chewing the food well so that it is easily digested.
(5) Only eating a light meal before chemotherapy.

If nausea and vomiting is a problem, patients must tell their chemotherapy nurse and doctor. Alternative antisickness treatment may be helpful.

Sore mouth (mucositis or stomatitis)

Some drugs damage the cells lining the mouth and cause soreness and ulceration. As patients may be prone to developing infections it is very important that they take great care of their mouth if it becomes sore.

Good mouth care includes (1) Regular brushing of teeth (up to 4 times per day) with a soft round bristle toothbrush. (2) Mouth washes after each brushing. A mixture of 1 teaspoon of baking soda to one cup of warm water may be used. Commercial mouth washes containing alcohol should be avoided. (3) using dental floss between the teeth as well as brushing. (4) If the soreness becomes severe or white patches develop in the mouth, patients should see their doctor as they may have thrush (an infection with a fungus called candida). This requires intensive treatment with antifungal mouth washes or lozenges in addition to the usual mouth care. (5) Avoid alcohol and spicy foods (including salt) that may cause a burning sensation. (6) Eat soft foods; try putting normal foods in a blender, and make sure there is plenty of gravy to moisten them.

The drugs that most commonly cause mucositis (Appendix A) are methotrexate, bleomycin, adriamycin, and daunomycin.

Diarrhoea

Diarrhoea is sometimes a problem. Doctors should be able to give medicines for this but patients may also help cope with it by, (1)

Eating warm foods rather than hot (hot food speeds up the bowel movements). (2) Avoiding foods high in fibre, these include raw fruits and vegetables, whole grain cereals and nuts. (3) Avoiding gassy foods such as cabbage, cauliflower, and baked beans. The drugs that most commonly cause diarrhoea are 5-fluorauracil and cis platin (Appendix A).

Bone marrow suppression or low blood count

The bone marrow is where the body makes the cells that circulate in the blood. Red blood cells prevent anaemia and carry oxygen around the body. White blood cells fight infections and the platelets help the blood to clot. Because the bone marrow cells that make these three types of blood cells are dividing rapidly (page 94) they are frequently damaged by chemotherapy. This damage is temporary, but it is common for the cells in the blood (measured by a blood count) to drop to low levels for a week or so after each treatment and doctors will ask for a blood count before each treatment to ensure that the patient's count is at a safe level to continue treatment. If the level of the white cells or platelets is too low, chemotherapy may be delayed a week or the dose of drugs reduced. If the patient has become anaemic (low red cells) a blood transfusion will be given.

- The amount that the blood counts drops depends very much on the intensity and type of treatment. Patients with a low white count should take precautions to help prevent an infection. (1) Avoid crowds or people with contagious diseases (those caught through close contact). (2) Take great care in cutting nails and caring for the cuticles. (3) Wear protective gloves if gardening or doing any dirty jobs. Despite this patients may still develop an infection as some of the normal bacteria (germs) living in the body may become aggressive and attack the body if its normal defence mechanisms are damaged. Patients developing the following symptoms *must* see their doctor quickly: (a) temperature (fever) over 100° Fahrenheit, (b) feeling hot or cold and shivering (rigors), (c) frequency and burning on passing urine, (d) cough, (e) diarrhoea for more than 2 days.

  Patients who have an infection whilst their blood count is low must see a doctor immediately as urgent and intensive antibiotic treatment in hospital is necessary. It is dangerous to ignore an infection whilst the blood count is low.

- Platelets (the clotting cells in the blood) may become low after treatment so that patients may bruise or bleed even with the slightest injury. Patients who have abnormal bleeding (nose bleeds, bleeding gums, blood in urine or faeces), or easy bruising or tiny red spots under the skin (bleeding spots called petechae) should contact their doctor immediately.

  A transfusion of platelets may be needed. These may need to be repeated over several days as the platelets (unlike red cells in a normal transfusion) only work for a short time. Patients whose platelets are low should:

    (1) Avoid injury and if they do cut themselves apply firm pressure with a clean cloth for several minutes. If this does not stop the bleeding they should call their doctor.
    (2) Do not garden.
    (3) Do not use any aspirin containing drugs (check *all* drugs labels for aspirin), as aspirin damages platelets.
    (4) Do not drink alcohol.

- Patients with a low red cell count are anaemic and may develop the following symptoms: (1) tiredness and irritability, (2) dizziness, especially on exertion or when standing up suddenly, (3) shortness of breath, (4) feeling cold. Patients with these symptoms should tell their doctor as a blood transfusion will make them feel much better if they are anaemic.

Hair loss

Cells in the hair follicles are dividing rapidly and may be affected by some types of chemotherapy. As a result scalp and body hair are comonly lost *temporarily* during treatment. Loss of hair is called alopecia. Losing one's hair is very upsetting and patients have to make a brave adjustment; some people like to cover their head whilst others prefer not to. Wigs are available on the National Health Service in Britain (it is advisable to order a wig at the start of treatment so that it can be matched to the patient's own hair) and some patients use a scarf or cap. Hair usually begins to fall out about 2–3 weeks after the first treatment and with two drugs (adriamycin and daunorubicin) the loss is complete, though it is variable with other drugs. The hair may start to grow back slightly during treatment and will gradually regrow after treatment. Often the new hair is thicker, curlier and sometimes darker or greyer than before. Although loss of scalp hair is most obvious other body hair including pubic hair is frequently lost. The drugs (Appendix A) that most commonly cause hair loss are: adriamycin and daunorubicin (nearly *always* cause temporary complete hair loss), cyclophosphamide, 5-FU, actinomycin D, vincristine, and VP16–213. Attempts to reduce hair loss with scalp tourniquets (a tight band round the head to reduce scalp blood flow) and by freezing the scalp have been partially successful but are still experimental techniques. It must be remembered that not all drugs cause hair loss and patients in doubt should ask their doctor.

Skin Effects

Allergic skin rashes may develop during treatment. These are usually red, raised itchy rashes which are often over much of the body. Doctors can give tablets to reduce the symptoms and will try to find out which drug caused the rash. Any drug can cause a rash but procarbazine (Appendix A) is the chemotherapy drug which most commonly causes allergic rashes.

Anticancer drugs may also irritate veins around the place where they were injected. This may be uncomfortable and there may be a red or dark line over the vein. Bleomycin (Appendix A) often causes increased skin pigmentation (tanning) which is most intense at pressure points so that the elbows are often pigmented, as are any scratch marks. Busulphan (Appendix A) may also cause some skin pigmentation.

Nail changes may occur with many drugs. Because of slowing of nail growth during each treatment there may be white lines in the nails corresponding with each treatment. Nails may also flake or break easily.

Some drugs may damage the skin and underlying tissues if allowed to leak from the vein when they are being injected. If this happens it usually causes pain and if patients feel any pain during an injection into a vein they must tell the nurse or doctor immediately so that the injection can be stopped. Even small amounts of drug that have leaked can cause a sore or ulcer which is very difficult to heal. The drugs (Appendix A) that can cause this side-effect are adriamycin, daunorubicin, actinomycin D, vincristine, vinblastine, and nitrogen mustard.

Nerves and muscles

Two drugs (vinblastine and vincristine – Appendix A) frequently affect nerves relaying sensation to the brain and nerves controlling muscles. The commonest side-effect is pins and needles (called paraesthesia) affecting the fingers and toes. Nearly all patients receiving these drugs will notice some effects. If the symptoms progress to affect the whole hand or foot or cause difficulty in holding small objects patients should tell their doctor. Weakness in the hands and legs can be caused by these drugs and it is important that the chemotherapy nurse or doctor knows of any muscle weakness as the dose of the drug needs to be reduced or the drug stopped because the weakness may become permanent if treatment is continued. 'Pins and needles' and minor muscle weakness usually clear up gradually over the first few months after treatment has stopped. Occasionally other drugs (especially cis platin) can cause similar symptoms, and patients should tell their doctor about any symptoms of this type as the drugs may need to be stopped.

Muscle weakness, by itself, is common after high doses of steroids (Appendix A); the weakness recovers when the drug is stopped but in a few patients may be quite marked.

Ovarian and testicular effects

Women having menstrual periods often develop irregular periods and possibly stop having periods altogether (amenorrhoea) during chemotherapy and menopausal symptoms (hot flushes, etc.) can occur as a result of treatment. When chemotherapy is stopped menstruation usually returns to normal and periods follow their previous pattern. Occasionally, when menstrual periods have stopped altogether during chemotherapy they may fail to return to normal. This usually happens in women over 30 years of age and the drugs appear to bring menopause on early. Despite abnormal periods during chemotherapy women may still become pregnant and they must use birth control methods. The 'pill' is not recommended and patients should discuss contraception with their doctor. Anticancer drugs can damage an unborn baby (page 105) and care to avoid pregnancy is *important*.

The eggs (ova) in the ovary are formed before birth and one matures with each menstrual cycle. The eggs are not damaged by the chemotherapy so that fertility may return to normal (provided that periods return) after the chemotherapy has stopped. Many women who have been treated with chemotherapy have subsequently become pregnant. The numbers of patients who do not have return of normal periods has not been carefully studied for each type of drug treatment, and women should discuss the possible effects on their fertility of the particular treatment that is planned. Reduced fertility is more common if chemotherapy has been given together with radiotherapy to the lower abdomen.

Chemotherapy in men is much more likely to damage the ability of the testis to make new sperm. Unlike the ovaries the testes are constantly making sperm and because the cells are dividing rapidly they are very susceptible to anticancer drugs. Not all drugs will damage the testes, the alkylating agents (Appendix A) are the main culprits, and some men remain fertile despite intensive chemotherapy. If the testes are severely damaged it is likely to be a permanent effect and the incidence of sterility is very high with certain drug combinations so that it is important that men discuss this with their doctor. Some hospitals have the facilities for storing sperm at very low temperatures (in liquid nitrogen), which allows the option of subsequent artificial insemination.

Although some patients may become sterile the chemotherapy should not interfere with their sex life. The hormones produced by the testes are not affected by chemotherapy though stress and tiredness and general malaise of the treatment may temporarily lessen desire (libido) for sex.

Chemotherapy in pregnancy

Chemotherapy can damage an unborn baby (foetus). The foetus is at most risk during the first three months and doctors usually advise a therapeutic abortion for any women treated with anticancer drugs during the first part of a pregnancy. Chemotherapy may sometimes be damaging later in pregnancy and these drugs are best avoided throughout pregnancy. Normal babies have been born occasionally to women who have received chemotherapy late in pregnancy. Patients with *any* reason to think that they may be pregnant before or during treatment must tell their doctor so that a pregnancy test can be arranged.

Effects on urine

Some drugs, notably adriamycin and daunorubicin (red), colour the urine for a few hours after treatment. Cyclophosphamide and a new related drug (Iphosphamide) may cause a chemical cystitis (inflammation of the bladder). The drug is broken down in the body into compounds which irritate the bladder when they are in large amounts in the urine. Because of this patients should increase their fluid intake (to at least 4 pints per day) for a day or two after treatment with these drugs. This has the effect of rapidly flushing the drug out of the bladder. The symptoms of cystitis are discomfort or burning on passing urine, increased frequency of passing urine and blood in the urine and any patient with these symptoms should contact their doctor immediately. The symptoms usually stop when drug treatment is finished but may become troublesome if it is continued or repeated.

Chemotherapy and other drugs

Some drugs may affect treatment (interact) with anticancer drugs. If you are taking any of the following drugs you should tell your doctor.

   Antibiotics
   Anticoagulants (drugs to thin the blood and prevent clots)
   Anticonvulsants (drugs to prevent seizures in epilepsy)
   Aspirin (check all patent medicines which may contain aspirin)
   Barbiturates (rarely used sleeping pills)
   Blood pressure tablets
   Diabetic drugs
   Diuretics (water tablets)
   Hormone pills (including contraceptive pills)
   Nasal sprays (decongestant)
   Sleeping pills
   Tranquillizers (Valium, etc)
   Immunizations or vaccines. Live vaccines (e.g. smallpox jab)
      should **never** be given to patients receiving anticancer drugs.
      Always tell your doctor that you are on chemotherapy before
      having an immunization.

Patients with any doubts about possible interactions between drugs they are taking should ask if they will 'react' with the chemotherapy drugs.

Increased risk of cancer

Many of the anticancer drugs are carcinogens (page 4), chemicals which can cause cancer, and patients treated with and cured by chemotherapy have a slightly increased risk of a second cancer. This risk is, however, small compared with the benefit of curative chemotherapy and is highest in patients receiving both chemotherapy and radiotherapy.

Other side-effects

Most of the side-effects discussed are general and patients must ask their doctor about any particular side-effects caused by individual drugs they may be receiving (see common side-effects of the drugs in Appendix A).

WHEN SHOULD PATIENTS CALL THEIR DOCTOR ABOUT SIDE-EFFECTS?

It is important to contact a doctor *early* if patients have *any* side-effects that worry them. Some complications can become serious if not treated promptly and correctly; others are much less important and patients can be reassured. Early contact with a doctor will reduce worry about symptoms and will identify the side-effects which require more urgent treatment.

EMOTIONAL EFFECTS

Undergoing cancer therapy is very stressful and highly emotional for most patients. Family and friends should understand that feelings like anger, depression, fear, and apathy are to be expected (see Chapter Nineteen on communication). In addition to the stresses of the treatment itself some drugs (particularly high dose steroids), can occasionally cause emotional upsets by themselves. Supportive therapy during this period is important and in addition to family and friends it is useful for patients to be able to discuss problems and fears with doctors and nurses, and perhaps a psychiatrist, or psychotherapist, if reaction to the diagnosis and treatment is especially emotionally traumatic. There really should be no stigma attached to these emotional problems; all patients have them to some degree. One of the most depressing features of treatment given in monthly cycles is that just as patients are getting back to normal the next treatment, with its attendant side-effects, comes around.

QUESTIONS TO ASK ABOUT CHEMOTHERAPY

  (1) Why is drug treatment necessary?
  (2) What are the aims of chemotherapy?
  (3) How are the drugs given?
  (4) Are there any immediate side-effects?
  (5) Do I need to go into hospital for treatment?
  (6) If not, can I drive home afterwards?
  (7) How often is the treatment given?
  (8) How long does each treatment take?
  (9) How many courses of treatment are planned? (If given, as tablets, continuously; what is the duration of treatment?)
(10) Are there any later side-effects (in particular does it affect fertility)?
(11) Should I take any special precautions before or after chemotherapy?
(12) How can I contact the hospital in case of worrying side-effects?

CHAPTER FIFTEEN

Quack remedies and unconventional treatments

To be told that one has cancer is a devastating experience; learning that it is uncurable is even worse. At such times patients naturally look anywhere for solace and many will turn to 'fringe' medicine or to 'new' techniques for which extravagant, unrealistic, and usually unproven claims are made.

Occasionally such searchs may be used subconsciously by the patient or his family to deny the reality and unpleasantness of what is happening. We all know of people especially children, who are dragged across the world to some 'specialist' who can apparently solve the problem. The cost of this adventure is often high in financial terms, physical distress, and dashed hopes. The wise physician will carefully consider the treatment being offered, the patient's and family's desires and will try to dissuade them from embarking on a hopeless course. If sensitively done most families will be grateful.

Unconventional medicine is most commonly used in the United States but is on the increase in Europe and the UK and they include the following:

- Laetril (also known as vitamin B_{17} or nitriloside). This is an extract of apricot stones (pits) containing cyanide. The cyanide is said to be released in cancer cells killing them. There is no scientific evidence to support the claims of Laetril despite its widespread use over more than two decades. Many patients have paid large sums of money for supplies of Laetril in the United States and at clinics in Mexico; but few if any, have been helped by it.

Some trials testing the usefulness of Laetril are in progress in the United States as there has been a very strong pressure to legalize the use of the drug (it has no drug licence). These trials show that it is useless so it should never be considered as treatment for curable tumours.

Laetril is not without side-effects and deaths from an overdose of the drug (containing cyanide) have occurred, especially in children who have mistaken them for sweets.

- Diet therapies. Special diets are a popular new way of trying to treat cancer and they are growing in popularity in England. There is no evidence that they can cause a tumour to shrink, but are not harmful provided they do not delay the conventional treatment of a curable tumour. They are also relatively inexpensive and most vitamins are not dangerous in large doses though vitamins A and D can be harmful in the large doses sometimes recommended.
- Another area of dubious therapy is the use of various enemas some of which use unusual substances such as coffee. They are of no proven value.
- Courses of special immunization and injections (such as material from animal placentas) are used by some practitioners. They can cause allergic reactions such as rashes, asthma, and fevers. They are dangerous and should be avoided.
- 'Cancer Centres' or clinics have been set up which provide some or all of these treatments. Often the standard of care and support in these centres is high, but they cannot cure cancer. Their success, however, does underline the failure of conventional medicine to support patients emotional and physical needs.

Any patient contemplating unconventional remedies should discuss it fully with their doctor. If there is a chance for cure with conventional treatment, even at the risk of side-effects, this should not be missed by opting for unconventional or unrecognized therapies.

As well as these 'treatments' for cancer, groups have stressed the importance of the mental approach to cancer. There is no doubt that a negative or defeatist attitude to cancer or any disease is bad. These groups say that by using a positive mental approach directed against a tumour cancer patients can cure their own tumour. For instance, patients are encouraged to try to shrink their cancer by imagining their own white cells eating the tumour. Getting patients to think optimistically and to help fight against cancer is good but telling them that if they think in the 'right' way they can shrink a cancer is more difficult. If the cancer does grow it only makes the patient feel that he has failed though he may still feel that he has helped with his own treatment. Cancers are not cured by the power of will alone though a constructive and determined frame of mind must be beneficial.

DO'S AND DONT'S OF CANCER QUACKERY

- Discuss it with your doctor
- Consider if those who claim to be cured are really cured.
- Is the treatment harmful?
- How much does it cost and will the person giving the treatment gain financially?
- Has anyone you know and *trust* had similar treatment or know about it?
- Has the treatment been tested scientifically. Reports or stories about 'wonder' cures cannot usually be relied on, however impressive.
- Go into any untested treatment with an open mind.

CHAPTER SIXTEEN

How are the common cancers treated?

The aim of this chapter is to outline the types of treatment used so that patients and relatives can discuss their own particular treatment more fully.

Cancer treatment is becoming an area of medicine that requires a team approach. In some tumours many medical skills (diagnostic x-ray, pathology, surgery, radiotherapy, and chemotherapy, etc.) are needed for good treatment and it is important that one doctor, working with others, makes all the final decisions.

Those tumours that are curable but need complicated management, should always be referred to a major cancer centre. However, if no useful treatment is available or if the curative treatment is simple then routine referral is not necessary. It is not possible to be dogmatic about which patients should be referred to special centres but the following tumours are examples of the type of tumour that benefit from expert treatment.

(1) Choriocarcinoma.
(2) Testicular teratomas.
(3) Leukaemias.
(4) All childhood tumours.
(5) Lymphomas.
(6) Hodgkin's disease.
(7) Sarcomas of bone and soft tissues.

Many of these tumours require a combination of surgery, radiotherapy or chemotherapy and are all potentially curable. The best chance of cure comes with the first treatment and it is important that the best care is given right from the start.

In this long chapter the various tumours are divided into groups by the system to which they belong, e.g. stomach is part of the gastrointestinal tract. Discussion includes sections on symptoms, diagnosis, and treatment; the treatment of tumours requiring longer discussion is summarized at the end of each section. The chapter has extensive cross-referencing and is best used together with the chapters on screening, investigation, surgery, radio-therapy, and chemotherapy. Space for notes on treatment has been left after each section.

GASTROINTESTINAL TRACT

Cancer of the stomach

Cancers of the stomach (Figure 27) have become less common in Western countries during the past forty years. In contrast, the incidence of this tumour is so high in Japan that a special screening programme has been started.

The stomach is the first part of the digestive tract which is in contact with food for a long time (up to 3 hours). It has, therefore, been suggested that substances (carcinogens) in some foods cause cancer. No particular food has been shown to be carcinogenic but diets high in smoked foods, salt fish, pickled vegetables, and grains have been suspected.

It is a disease of late middle age (50–70 years) and is more common in heavy drinkers and in sufferers of pernicious anaemia (lack of vitamin B_{12}) but no other predisposing factors are known.

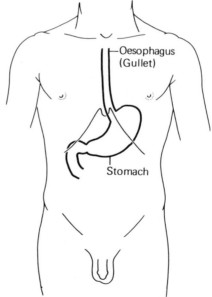

Figure 27 Diagrammatic representation of the upper gastrointestinal tract showing the position of the stomach

SYMPTOMS

The symptoms of stomach cancer are similar to those of an ulcer and include:

- Indigestion or upper abdominal pains; these may be helped by antacids, by eating, or by drinking milk.
- Vomit containing blood.
- Loss of appetite or weight.

Unfortunately many stomach cancers do no produce symptoms till they are quite far advanced. Any indigestion that does not clear quickly should be taken seriously and the advice of a doctor sought.

DIAGNOSIS

Patients with persistent upper abdominal pains or any of the above symptoms should have investigations to find out the cause. In many cases cancer is not found, but it is important to be sure.
The tests used include:

- A barium meal (page 44). In this test a white liquid, which shows up on an x-ray and outlines the stomach, is swallowed.
- Gastroscopy (page 74). In this test a special flexible instrument is swallowed and is used to look into the stomach. If a suspicious area is seen, a small piece (a biopsy) can be taken for examination under a microscope.
- Other tests may include a chest x-ray, blood tests and if a cancer is found a liver scan (page 63) or possibly a CT body scan (page 59).

TREATMENT

Unfortunately, stomach cancer is frequently not diagnosed till it is quite advanced and many patients die of the tumour.

Surgery

(Chapter Twelve) is the most important treatment and may be curative in some patients whose disease is at an early stage. Operations for stomach cancer may require removal of all or a large part of the stomach and its local lymph glands (page 36). Patients who have had such an operation (radical or total gastrectomy) usually require a special diet consisting of regular small amounts of foods that are high in protein and fat but low in sugar. Regular injections of vitamin B_{12} may also be necessary. It is usually necessary to make a vertical incision (cut) over the upper abdomen and following the operation tubes or drains may be temporarily left in the abdomen to remove any blood or fluid. Patients will be up soon after the operation and should be able to leave hospital after 10–14 days.

Unfortunately in many patients the tumour is too far advanced for such an operation to be helpful.

Radiotherapy

(Chapter Thirteen) is not routinely used for the treatment of stomach cancer though it may be useful in dealing with symptoms such as pain caused by secondary spread.

Chemotherapy

(Chapter Fourteen) although some drugs are helpful in stomach cancer they cannot cure advanced disease. The chemotherapy most commonly used is the drug 5-FU given alone though recent work has suggested that combinations of two or three drugs may be more active (these often include adriamycin or mitomycin C – Appendix A). About a quarter of patients treated with chemotherapy have a useful response but only a few patients respond for a long time. In cases of advanced stomach cancer there are three possible approaches to the tumour: (1) No anticancer treatment, apart from therapy for specific symptoms, (2) a simple treatment with few side-effects (such as 5-FU) may be used, and (3) patients may be included in a trial of combination chemotherapy. There are no clear rules for the treatment of advanced stomach cancer but it is probably best to avoid drug combinations in patients who are generally unwell because of their tumour. Combination chemotherapy remains unproven and ideally should be used only in trials testing its usefulness (page 321). In patients with a small tumour, trials of combination chemotherapy (adjuvant therapy, page 143) after surgery are being run but the results yet do not support the routine use of such treatment.

SUMMARY OF TREATMENT OF STOMACH CANCER

(1) Stomach cancer is becoming less common in Western countries and screening is not helpful.
(2) Unexplained indigestion or ulcer symptoms should be investigated.
(3) Surgery is potentially curative but most patients already have extensive disease that cannot be treated by surgery.
(4) Radiotherapy may be used to control symptoms.
(5) Drug therapy may consist of 5-FU alone or drugs in combination but is only useful in about a quarter of patients.
(6) Adjuvant chemotherapy is not of proven use and trials continue.

Notes

Pancreas

The pancreas is a gland that lies below the stomach and alongside the first part of the bowel (Figure 28) and produces digestive enzymes and insulin. The digestive enzymes get into the bowel by a small tube called the pancreatic duct.

The pancreas lies deep in the abdomen and tumours of this gland are rarely diagnosed at an early stage when they are curable.

SYMPTOMS

There are no early symptoms and patients rarely notice anything wrong until the tumour is advanced and has invaded nearby organs. The main symptoms are:

- Pain in the upper abdomen and frequently in the back.
- Weight loss.

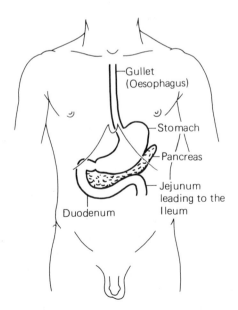

Figure 28 Diagrammatic representation of the upper gastrointestinal tract showing the position of the pancreas

- Loss of appetite.
- Jaundice (the accumulation of yellow bile pigment in the body which causes a yellow appearance of the whites of the eyes and the skin).

DIAGNOSIS

As the pancreas is such a deep-seated organ it is often difficult to make the diagnosis of pancreatic cancer. The usual tests include:

- Barium meal (page 44) to see if the pancreas is enlarged and is pressing on the duodenum (see Figure 28).
- Ultrasound examination (page 59) of the upper abdomen to see if there is a lump in the region of the pancreas.
- CT body scan (page 59) will also show if there is a lump in this area.
- Endoscopy (page 76), including ERCP, allows the doctor to examine the pancreatic duct as it enters the bowel and to pass a fine tube into the duct so that some contrast dye can be injected and an x-ray picture taken.
- Occasionally an arteriogram (page 54) may be done to outline the blood vessels in the gland.

As it may be difficult to be certain of the diagnosis of pancreatic cancer it is often necessary to do several of these tests.

TREATMENT

Unfortunately, in most patients the tumour is too far advanced at diagnosis for there to be a hope of cure but treatment to control the tumour or relieve symptoms can be given.

Surgery

(Chapter Twelve) If the tests discussed above suggest a pancreatic cancer an exploratory abdominal operation (a laparotomy) is usually performed. A biopsy should be taken to prove the diagnosis if cancer is suspected and a careful assessment for any possible spread in the abdomen is then made. In most patients tumour is found beyond the pancreas and surgery is palliative (page 81), being designed to prevent further symptoms. The main aim is to prevent obstruction of the bile duct (this would cause jaundice) or of the bowel. Occasionally the tumour appears to be only in the pancreatic gland and a surgical operation to remove the pancreas may be planned. This operation (a Whipples procedure or radical pancreatectomy) is technically difficult even when done by an experienced surgeon.

Some surgeons doubt that a Whipples procedure is ever very helpful but it may be useful when done on very carefully selected patients with small tumours and who are in good general health. After a Whipples procedure patients will, like diabetics, require insulin replacement therapy.

Radiation therapy

(Chapter Thirteen) Radiotherapy may be useful in treating some of the symptoms of pancreatic cancer but cure is very unlikely. Trials of radiotherapy in the treatment of pancreatic cancer are being run at present.

Chemotherapy

(Chapter Fourteen) Anticancer drug therapy is of limited value as only about a quarter of the patients respond and the responses are only temporary. 5-FU is the most frequently used drug but several other drugs may be used (including adriamycin and mitomycin C – Appendix A). Combination drug therapy should ideally only be used in trials (page 321) as its role remains undefined. Although most patients do not benefit from chemotherapy occasional good responses do occur.

It is important if a pancreatic cancer is found to discuss the aims of treatment at the outset. Cure is only occasionally possible and treatment is usually designed to prevent symptoms and prolong life.

SUMMARY OF THE TREATMENT OF PANCREATIC CANCER

(1) Pancreatic cancer is usually found at a late stage.
(2) It may be difficult to make the diagnosis.
(3) Surgery is usually palliative (designed to prevent symptoms).

(4) Occasionally radical removal of the pancreas may be curative.
(5) Radiotherapy is only useful for controlling symptoms.
(6) Chemotherapy is not very active in this tumour. Combination chemotherapy has shown early promise but is best used in trials.

Notes

Liver cancer

There is often confusion between cancers that have developed elsewhere, the bowel for example, and spread to the liver and cancers developing in the liver itself. Spread to the liver (secondary cancer) is common whilst primary liver cancers are rare in Western countries though interestingly they are common in parts of Africa and the Far East. Only cancers *developing* in the liver should normally be called liver cancer and this section only deals with these tumours.

Some liver cancers may be caused by exposure to chemicals and vinyl chloride is known to have caused some tumours. Some male hormones (testosterone) and the oral contraceptive pill can cause liver tumours though many of these are benign, it should, however, be remembered that this risk is small. Liver cancer is also more common in people who have alcoholic cirrhosis and over half the cases of liver cancer in the West are associated with cirrhosis.

SYMPTOMS

These are often vague and include:

- Weakness.
- Loss of appetite.
- Abdominal discomfort or pain.
- Bloated abdomen.

The diagnosis may be complicated by an underlying cirrhosis which can cause similar symptoms itself.

DIAGNOSIS

A biopsy of this liver is usually necessary (page 68). The optimal area to be biopsied may be shown by examining the liver with:

- Liver scan (page 63).
- Liver ultrasound (page 59).

TREATMENT

Unfortunately, the outlook is usually very poor. The only chance for cure depends on the rare finding of a cancer localized to one part of the liver. If this is the case then surgery to remove part of the liver, if the patient is fit enough, is attempted. This type of surgery should, preferably, only be done by a surgeon experienced in this field.

Radiation or chemotherapy can be given to the majority of patients (95 per cent) who cannot undergo surgery. Treatment should be designed to control symptoms and unfortunately many patients die within one year.

Notes

124

Cancer of the oesophagus (gullet)

The oesophagus is the tube that connects the mouth to the stomach (Figure 29). Rhythmic contractions of muscles in the wall of the oesophagus pass food and liquid into the stomach when swallowing.

Certain countries have a very high incidence of this cancer which is probably caused by cancer producing substances (carcinogens) in the environment. Among countries with a high incidence are Iran, Japan, and Finland. Japanese who go to live in the United States and who eat an American diet have a lower incidence of oesophageal cancer and for this reason it is thought that the tumour, may be caused by certain types of food.

In the West the most important predisposing factor is probably heavy alcohol use. The tumour may also occur in patients with other chronic and long-term benign conditions affecting the oesophagus.

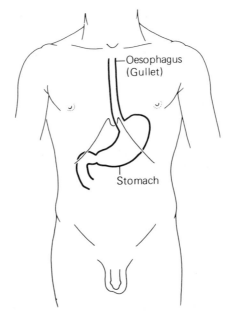

Figure 29 Diagrammatic representation of the upper gastrointestinal tract showing the course of the oesophagus (gullet)

These include: (1) the Plummer-Vinson syndrome which is a condition in young women where there is anaemia, difficulty in swallowing, and a web of tissue in the oesophagus. It is usually improved or cured by an adequate diet and iron supplements. The syndrome may also be known as the Kelly–Patterson or Sideropenic syndrome. (2) Achalasia, which is the loss of the normal rhythmic contractions of the gullet that aid swallowing, results in relaxation of the oesophageal walls and a ballooning of the oesophagus which contains fluid and undigested food particles. The resulting chronic inflammation predisposes to cancer. Operations can be used to correct achalasia. (3) Cancer is also more common in patients who have a stricture of the gullet caused by swallowing caustic liquids.

Routine screening is not justified in Western countries, but may be of value in those at high risk, though it has not been tested in such patients.

SYMPTOMS

This is a tumour that usually causes symptoms late in its course. The commonest complaints include:

- Difficulty in swallowing. This is initially on eating solids and later on swallowing fluids. This difficulty is often intermittent but is progressive.
- Pain in the chest or back.
- Weight loss.
- Anaemia caused by oozing loss of blood from the tumour.
- If the obstruction is severe, vomiting which is often blood-stained may occur.

DIAGNOSIS

This is usually straightforward and is made by x-ray and direct visual examination using an endoscope (Chapter Eleven). The test used are:

- Barium swallow (page 44).
- Oesophagoscopy using a flexible gastroscope (page 74). If a tumour is seen a biopsy (a small specimen of tissue) will be taken for examination under a microscope.

In patients found to have a tumour additional tests include:

- Chest x-ray
- Liver scan (page 63) or ultrasound (page 59)
- Blood tests of liver function.

TREATMENT

Unfortunately the tumour is usually at an advanced stage when the diagnosis is made so that curative surgery is often not possible. In addition only a quarter of tumours are in the lower part of the oesophagus where it is easier to perform an operation.

Surgery (Chapter Twelve)

Surgical removal of cancers of the lower third of the oesophagus is still technically difficult and only rarely cures patients. When it can be performed it restores normal swallowing. If on examination the tumour is not too big or fixed then a surgeon can remove the tumour and bring the stomach up into the chest and reconnect it to the upper part of the oesophagus. This is a major operation that is performed by a thoracic (chest) surgeon.

For tumours of the upper and middle parts of the oesophagus surgery is even more difficult. Operations designed to remove the tumour and then to bring part of the large bowel into the chest to reconnect the two ends of the oesophagus are occasionally done. The risk of complications and likelihood of death during or shortly after the operation are appreciable, and this sort of operation should only be considered in carefully selected cases where cure is the aim. This operation requires an incision (cut) over the chest and abdomen and a long recovery period is usually required. When an operation on the chest is performed drains are left in the chest for a few days to remove air or fluid.

Radiation therapy

(Chapter Thirteen) Radiotherapy can be useful palliative therapy (treatment for symptoms) in oesophageal cancer. It is the usual treatment for cancers of the upper oesophagus but may also be used for advanced cancers of the lower oesophagus.

Radiotherapy is given for 4 or 5 days each week for a total of 4–6 weeks. The first visit to the department is spent planning the individual treatment for the patient. Side-effects include:

- Some nausea.
- Loss of appetite.
- Irritation and reddening of the skin over the area being treated.
- Soreness on swallowing.

Radiotherapy is sometimes used together with surgery.

Chemotherapy

(Chapter Fourteen) Although the tumour may spread to the liver, lungs and bone there are, unfortunately, no useful drugs in oesophageal cancer and routine chemotherapy is not recommended though trials of experimental drug therapy continue.

PALLIATIVE TREATMENT

As patients with oesophageal cancer cannot swallow special ways of overcoming this have been designed. If a tumour is very advanced when first seen or if tumour comes back a special plastic tube may be pushed through the tumour opening up the oesophagus.

This is done at a minor operation and dramatically relieves symptoms, allows normal eating and in advanced cases is of great help.

SUMMARY OF TREATMENT OF OESOPHAGEAL CANCER

(1) Screening is of no value except possibly in those with conditions predisposing to the tumour.
(2) It is usually in an advanced stage at diagnosis.
(3) Surgery is rarely curative but is helpful in selected cases. Operations on the lower third are technically easier.
(5) Chemotherapy is ineffective and is best avoided unless new active drugs are found.
(6) The insertion of a plastic tube through the cancer may give very effective relief of symptoms.

Notes

Large bowel (colon or rectum) cancer

Cancer of the large bowel or lower intestine is very probably a problem associated with diet. In those countries where the people eat little fibre (roughage) but a lot of animal fats, protein, and refined sugar, the incidence is high, compared with that in places where plenty of fibre and little refined sugar or meat is eaten.

Diets low in fibre result in small stools and a slow transit time through the intestine. It has been suggested that the risk of cancer is higher if cancer causing substances (carcinogens, page 4) in the stool are in contact with the bowel wall for a long time and this is more likely to happen if transit is slow. As additional support for this theory some studies have suggested that bacteria in the bowel can break down animal fats to produce carcinogens.

The way our Western diet appears to increase our risk of colon cancer is not proven, but a move towards a diet including more roughage and less animal fats and protein has been recommended by some doctors.

The treatment of large bowel cancer is more likely to be successful the earlier a tumour is discovered and because of this efforts to screen for bowel cancer have been made. Although routine examination of stools for blood is done in the United States, it is rarely used in Europe. The usefulness of large scale screening programmes remains doubtful but in those patients at *high risk* (page 13) routine screening of stools for blood together with a regular examination of the lower bowel may be advisable. Conditions that may predispose to bowel cancer are discussed in Chapter four.

The colon is a muscular tube that starts at the right side of the abdomen and is about 1.5m long and ends at the anus. Descriptively it is divided into several parts as shown in Figure 30.

SYMPTOMS AND INVESTIGATIONS

The main presenting symptoms of large bowel cancer are:

- Blood in the stools.
- Feeling of fullness or pain in the rectum.

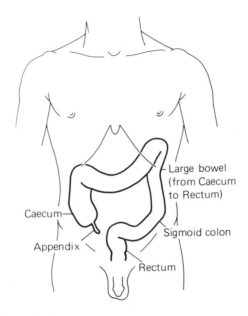

Figure 30 Diagrammatic representation of the course of the large bowel

- Difficulty in evacuating the bowel.
- Persistent constipation or diarrhoea.
- Thin stringy stools.
- Pain in the lower abdomen.
- Anaemia (due to lack of iron) without explanation.

Nearly all colon cancers bleed and the approach to a patient with symptoms that suggest a cancer includes:

- Examination of the stool for blood.
- A rectal examination and general physical examination.
- Sigmoidoscopy (page 72) to look into the lower bowel and obtain a biopsy if possible.
- Barium enema (page 46) and possibly colonoscopy and biopsy (page 73).

If a cancer is found then a chest x-ray, blood tests, and liver ultrasound (page 59) or isotope scan (page 63) should be done before surgery is planned. If these show spread of tumour it may alter surgical management.

TREATMENT

Surgery

(Chapter Twelve) Surgical removal of the tumour cures up to half of patients with colon cancer and is the most important treatment. During and after surgery the extent of tumour spread in the bowel is carefully looked at as the likelihood of cure is closely related to the degree of spread or 'stage' of the cancer (Chapter ten). The staging sytem used for large bowel cancer is known as the 'Dukes classification'. If the cancer is confined to the lining (mucosa) of the bowel (Dukes' A) the chance of cure is very high. If the cancer has invaded into the muscle wall of the bowel (Dukes' B) the chances are intermediate whilst if the tumour has spread to local lymph nodes (Dukes' C) they are least good.

The type of operation used to remove the tumour varies from patient to patient. If the cancer is very close to the anus then it is impossible to remove the tumour and to join the ends of the bowel together, as incontinence will follow the operation. In such cases a colostomy (page 328) is performed. In this operation the rectum is removed and the colon is brought through the lower abdominal wall which is covered with a special bag to collect stool. It is, of course, always difficult for patients to adjust to the idea of a colostomy but, most patients after initial worries adjust well and lead a normal life. Special nurses (stoma nurses) trained in the care of colostomies help with the early adjustment and colostomy associations (see Appendix D) in Britain and the United States have volunteers (usually with colostomies themselves) who will help new patients.

Most patients with bowel cancer do not require a colostomy as the bowel can be joined together when the tumour has been removed. Fewer patients have a colostomy these days as new techniques for joining the bowel together allow operations nearer to the lower end of the rectum. Occasionally patients only develop symptoms when a cancer of the bowel causes obstruction. In such cases a surgeon may initially perform a colostomy even though the tumour is not near the anus. After the effects of the obstruction have settled down (usually some months) the colostomy is often taken away and the ends of the bowel are joined together again.

Whether or not a colostomy is necessary the very best chance of curing this cancer lies with surgery. The technique of the operation depends on where the tumour is and patients should discuss which type of operation is being planned for them.

Radiation therapy

(Chapter Thirteen) Recent trials have suggested that in patients at increased risk of tumour recurrence (Dukes' stage B or C) radiation may reduce the frequency of relapse if the tumour arises in the last part of the colon (sigmoid colon) or rectum (Figure 30). The side-effects of radiotherapy include diarrhoea, loss of appetite, and tiredness. Treatment lasts about four weeks and is given 4 to 5 times each week, the first visit being used to plan the treatment for the individual patient. Radiotherapy has only been used in this way recently and may be given before or after an operation; it is not routinely used for tumours of the rest of the large bowel.

Chemotherapy

(Chapter Fourteen) Drugs have been used to treat advanced bowel cancer for a number of years. One drug (5-fluorouracil – Appendix A) has been the mainstay of treatment and there is no evidence that adding other drugs to 5-FU improve its activity. Unfortunately only about one in every five patients has a useful response to treatment, though 5-FU is relatively free of side-effects (Appendix A) and is well tolerated by most patients.

As the response to chemotherapy is not good it is not routinely used as adjuvant therapy (page 143) after surgery. Trials of adjuvant treatment are taking place but until it is proven that this treatment is useful it should be avoided.

In some patients with metastatic spread of cancer a course of 5-FU chemotherapy is warranted. If there is no response after several courses further treatment is not helpful. There are few good alternative drugs though some patients may be treated with new drugs in trials (Chapter Twenty); unfortunately, none look promising at the moment.

SUMMARY

(1) People at *high risk* of colon cancer should probably have routine screening tests. Those at no obvious increased risk

should seek medical advice if they develop any of the symptoms of large bowel cancer. Programmes of screening of normal populations continue but are uproven.

(2) Surgery is the mainstay of treatment and is curative in about half of patients. Patients having a colostomy should receive help from stoma nurses and if necessry local colostomy groups.

(3) Radiation therapy with surgery may be helpful in cancers of the last part of the bowel. Treatment may be given before or after the surgery.

(4) Chemotherapy is not very helpful for this tumour. The most useful drug, 5-FU, is relatively free of side-effects and combinations of drugs are best avoided. Adjuvant chemo-therapy is being tested but should not be given outside trials.

Notes

===================== BREAST =====================

Breast cancer is the commonest cancer in women living in the Western world. Early diagnosis is important as a tumour confined to the breast can be cured. Screening for breast cancer (Chapter Seven) remains unproven except for those at high risk of developing a tumour, however periodic self-examination does make sense.

Women using self-examination (page 26) should be shown how to do it by someone experienced in the technique and if this cannot be arranged locally there are cancer organizations that can help (Appendix D). Self-examination should be done seven days after each period or in women after the menopause on the same day each month. Recommendations for mammography (a special breast x-ray) are discussed in the section on screening. The anatomy of the breast and the ways cancer may spread to lymph nodes is shown in Figure 31.

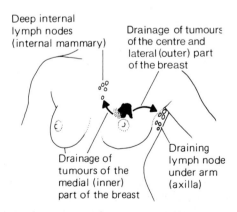

Figure 31 The routes of spread of breast cancer to lymph nodes

WHAT TO DO ABOUT A BREAST LUMP

Despite the apprehension that women feel on finding a breast lump it is much better to see a doctor quickly. Most lumps are not cancer at all and are harmless but this can only be decided by an experienced doctor. Women who have had previous harmless lumps should not ignore a new lump – all lumps should be examined. General practitioners should refer all patients with a breast lump to a breast clinic or to those experienced in the care of breast disease and if a general practitioner takes no action about a lump the patient should ask for a second opinion; even experienced breast surgeons cannot be sure a lump is benign without a biopsy. At the breast clinic patients, who are found to have a breast lump on examination, may have a mammogram (special x-ray of the breast – page 44) as the appearance of the lump in this test can help the doctor to decide on further management. All patients, however, should have a biopsy if there is a persistent firm lump. Cystic (fluid filled) lumps may be drained by sucking out the fluid with a syringe and needle. The fluid is then examined under a microscope to make sure that there are no malignant cells.

Some surgeons will do a breast biopsy under general anaesthetic and ask a pathologist to examine the tissue immediately (a frozen section) and if cancer is present will go on to perform a mastectomy (removal of the breast). Recently surgeons have begun to perform a biopsy, often under local anaesthetic, as a minor operation in a day ward. The biopsy tissue is examined by a pathologist after slower routine processing (this technique is more reliable than a frozen section) and if cancer is found a formal cancer operation is performed when the situation has been discussed with the patient. Such a biopsy may take the form of a small operation to remove the lump or the use of a special needle (True-cut) to remove a piece of the lump after a local anaesthetic has been given.

The major advantage of such an approach is that the need for, and surgical technique of any cancer operation can be fully explained and agreed with the patient before it is done. There is no disadvantage in waiting for the result of a biopsy and many breast units now use this approach. Patients should be given the choice of this type of delayed operation if they request it. Many patients find it helpful to have a chance of adjusting to the new situation before undergoing a mastectomy and in those patients whose lump is not cancer (*the majority*) they will not have to suffer the agony of anticipating waking from the anaesthetic to find their breast gone.

TREATMENT

If the lump is malignant the care of breast cancer involves a team of doctors experienced in various branches of medicine and many centres have breast clinics that bring these doctors together. Although there have been standard treatments in the past there are now several areas of controversy. Patients should discuss the treatment options so that they know the advantages and disadvantages of each form of treatment. Although the main controversies are covered in this chapter, it is a complex field and patients should take the opportunity to talk to their doctor about their own treatment.

Surgery

(Chapter Twelve) The usual operation for cancer of the breast has long been a Halstead Radical Mastectomy. This operation is disfiguring, as in addition to removal of the breast and lymph glands under the arm, a major part of the muscles on the front of the chest are removed. There is no evidence that this extensive operation is any better than operations not including removal of muscle.

A more modern and acceptable alternative operation is a modified radical or simple mastectomy. Whichever technique is

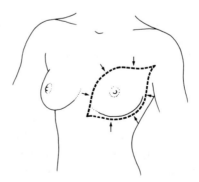

Figure 32 The type of incision (cut) used for the surgical removal of a breast (mastectomy)

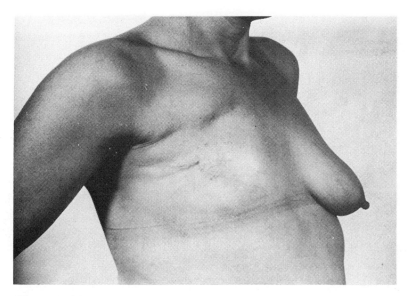

Figure 33 The scar left by the surgical removal of a breast (mastectomy)

used (there are minor technical differences) an incision (cut) is made and the breast and associated tissue (usually including the lymph nodes under the arm) are removed (Figure 32). The incision is stitched so that a single scar remains (Figure 33). A suction drain is often left in the wound immediately after the operation to prevent fluid accumulating under the scar; these tubes are removed after a few days. Although the breast is sensitive, post-operative pain is not usually severe and is well controlled by pain medicines. Physiotherapy is given after the operation to ensure that the shoulder does not get stiff and patients should be out of bed the day after the operation and the stitches are removed at 7–10 days, the patient is usually able to go home within one week.

Before leaving hospital patients should be given a light-weight breast prosthesis (artificial breast) to wear in the first few weeks after the operation. This restores the normal breast outline but does not exert pressure on the scar. Later the patient is supplied with a permanent breast prosthesis (Figure 34); patients should be helped in their choice and some hospitals now have specialist

138

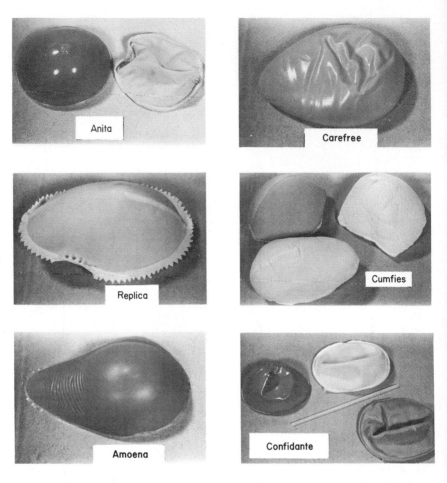

Figure 34 Different types of artificial breasts (prosthesis) currently used

mastectomy nurses. A suitable comfortable bra is also important and despite understandable early anxiety many patients are able to wear low cut dresses and swim suits if they have a properly fitted prosthesis and choose their clothes sensibly (Figure 35).

Following a mastectomy there is inevitably a deep sense of personal loss and many patients require time to adjust to the situation. The time required for adjustment varies considerably and is influenced not only by the patient's personality but also by

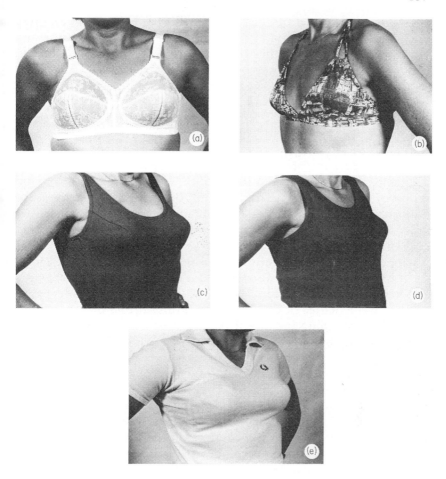

Figure 35 A woman who has had a mastectomy wearing various clothes with a prosthesis: (a) bra, (b) bikini, (c) one-piece swim suit, (d) sweater, (e) sports shirt

the care and understanding she receives from the hospital and her family.

Women who have had a mastectomy can lead an active sex life. Sexual difficulties can occur but should not always be blamed purely on the mastectomy – such difficulties are not uncommon at times of stress and anxiety. Support at times of emotional difficulty can be provided by breast clinics and groups such as the

Mastectomy Association (page 355) will give help. Women often do not complain of anxiety and depression to their doctor and mastectomy nurses or other trained nurses can be very helpful in identifying and discussing problems with patients. If expert guidance and counselling is needed this can be given by most breast clinics.

Other operations

Surgery to preserve the shape and appearance of the breast is also available. It is called a lumpectomy or quadrantectomy and removes some of the tissue around the cancer but leaves the majority of the normal breast. Such an operation is followed by radiation therapy to the remaining breast tissue to kill any cancer cells that may have been left behind. Cosmetic results can be good if patients are selected carefully; the operation is most successful if the lump is small and the normal breast is of at least moderate size.

Although many doctors will not recommend this type of operation the degree of conflict surrounding breast preservation is shown by the ruling in several American states that patients *must* be offered this option. Until clinical trials (page 321) have shown how good such an approach is, many surgeons will feel that the operation is second best as it may lower the chance of cure. There is, however, no doubt that in selected patients it allows the normal breast to be preserved and some hospitals have reported results as good as conventional surgery when patients are selected carefully. Many surgeons in addition to the removal of the cancer (by lumpectomy) remove lymph nodes from under the arm using a separate incision. This will not lessen the cosmetic effect and is useful in helping to decide if any further treatment is necessary (see section on chemotherapy, page 143).

This type of surgical approach *together* with radiotherapy is a valid alternative to a mastectomy in selected patients and women with breast cancer should discuss the advantages and disadvantages with their doctor. Lumpectomy without radiotherapy is, however, unacceptable.

Radiotherapy (Chapter Thirteen)

Following a conventional mastectomy many patients in the past received radiotherapy to the area of the breast and its local lymph nodes. This reduces the risk of the cancer recurring locally but has no effect on the survival of patients. Recently many radiotherapists have not felt that routine post-operative radiotherapy is justified though this remains controversial. For those cancers (the minority) arising in the inner (medial) side of the breast there is some agreement that radiotherapy may be useful. Women should discuss the advantages and disadvantages of post-operative radiotherapy if such therapy is suggested. Radiotherapy to the remaining normal breast should be routine for women having lumpectomy or other operation designed to conserve the breast.

• If radiotherapy is to be given, the first visit to the department is spent 'planning' the treatment. This consists of designing a personal treatment programme that is suited to the individual patient. When treatment starts it is usually given for 4 or 5 days each week and will last about 4 or 5 weeks. Because of the type of treatment given and the particular shape of the chest there may be some soreness of the chest wall for a short period. This is particularly common if a mastectomy has been done.

• If a tumour is large when a patient first sees her doctor or if the skin of the breast is involved it is often not useful to perform a mastectomy and x-ray therapy alone may be used. This treatment may include the use of radioactive wires (implanted during an operation under anaesthetic – page 91) for a few days. Such treatment may vary considerably from patient to patient and should be discussed with the radiotherapist.

• Radiation therapy is also used to treat recurrence of breast cancer. Radiotherapy is particularly useful for getting rid of pain caused by deposits of cancer in bone and is helpful in controlling tumour recurring on the chest wall at the site of the mastectomy operation.

CHEMOTHERAPY AND HORMONE THERAPY
(Chapter Fourteen)

• Hormone therapy has been used to treat breast cancer since the last century. It was originally shown that surgical removal of the ovaries (oophorectomy) caused shrinkage of breast cancer in about one-third of patients. Since then removal of the ovaries has been the standard first treatment if breast cancer recurs. Around one-third of patients have tumours whose growth is partly controlled by hormones and these are the ones that regress when the ovaries (which produces the hormone oestrogen) are removed. In the past few years it has become possible to identify the patients whose tumours are hormonally responsive. Tissue removed from the cancer is examined in the laboratory and levels of 'receptors' of oestrogen and progesterone can be measured. If these 'receptors' are present over two-thirds of the patients respond to removal of the ovaries; if they are absent virtually none respond.

• Although removal of the ovaries is still regarded as the best initial treatment for recurrent breast cancer by many doctors, new drug treatments can have similar effects. Hormone drug treatments have been used for many years but have had side-effects that have limited their use. Tamoxifen (also known as Novaldex) is a drug that blocks the effects of oestrogen (produced in the ovary) and it is probably as effective as removing the ovaries. It has few side-effects and many doctors now use it instead of an operation to remove the ovaries. The advantage of avoiding an operation is obvious, especially when it is remembered that many patients may not respond to the operation. Hormone receptors are frequently measured on tissue taken at the original mastectomy and the results can be used to predict if a patient will respond to hormonal treatment later. The chances that a tumour will respond can be improved from 30 per cent to between 60 per cent and 80 per cent if patients are selected according to the receptor information.

• Patients who have responded well to one hormonal treatment and then have tumour grow back are also likely to respond to different hormone therapy. This hormonal treatment may be totally different to the first one, but it seems that it is the change of the hormones in the tumour that slows its growth – indeed just stopping one hormonal treatment may cause shrinkage in the size of tumour.

Tamoxifen is known as an antioestrogen, other hormonal drugs that may be used include oestrogen-like drugs, progesterones and androgens (male hormones). Oestrogens may cause vaginal bleeding, retention of fluid, and clotting in veins. Androgens often induce changes in the body so that it becomes more male in appearance (virilization); the voice deepens and facial hair may grow. Both of these types of drug have been used extensively but their side-effects are a real problem and since the introduction of tamoxifen they are only used when other hormonal treatments have stopped working. Drugs which stop the adrenal glands working normally are also used. The adrenals produce a variety of hormones including cortisone and aminoglutethamide, a drug which stops the adrenal producing hormones, is always given together with prednisone (cortisone) tablets. Aminoglutethamide often causes temporary skin rashes or sleepiness, but if the tablets are continued these effects wear off and the dose can gradually be increased over 3–6 weeks.

In the past, patients who have responded to removal of the ovaries have been shown to respond to removal of the adrenals (adrenalectomy) or pituitary gland. Some patients who responded to oophorectomy have a second response to adrenalectomy and then a third response to removal of the pituitary gland. This sequence of operations is now less popular and drugs are being used instead of operations. The number of possible hormonal manoeuvres (operatons or drugs) is very complicated and it is important that patients discuss the treatment that is being planned. It is clear, however, that for those patients who do respond to hormones the quality of the response and its length is usually better than other types of therapy.

Chemotherapy is the use of drugs that kill cancer cells. As discussed in Chapter Fourteen, all anticancer drugs have side-effects and they are often not used for the initial therapy of recurrent breast cancer; hormonal treatments are considered first unless it is known that the tumour does not contain hormone receptors. Chemotherapy may, however, be used following mastectomy when all tumour has apparently been removed; this is known as adjuvant therapy.

Adjuvant therapy (therapy which is given in addition to the primary removal of a cancer – page 369)

About half of the patients having a mastectomy have a recurrence of breast cancer within ten yers. The risk of recurrent tumour is highest in those who are found to have cancer in lymph nodes removed at mastectomy. Because of the higher risk in these patients adjuvant drug therapy has been tested in clinical trials both in the United States and Europe. Despite the enthusiasm that has surrounded the introduction of adjuvant chemotherapy it is too early to be *sure* of the long term results. Breast cancer is unusual in that disease recurrence can occur up to ten or more years after mastectomy. Because of this it is important to wait for long follow-up of adjuvant trials before we can be certain that they improve the patient's chance of survival instead of just delaying the relapse.

Results, so far, suggest the following conclusions amongst patients found to have lymph nodes involved at mastectomy (node positive).

1. For women before or at their menopause there is a definite delay in tumour recurrence and a modest increase in survival of the whole group of patients. It should be remembered, however, that not all of these patients were going to relapse or die of breast cancer even if they did not receive adjuvant therapy.

2. In older women, past the menopause, there is also a definite delay in recurrence but it is more difficult to show that survival is better in those receiving adjuvant chemotherapy. All trials show a trend in this direction but in none is it very large.

Trials have compared the effects of adjuvant therapy in women with a similar group of women receiving no adjuvant chemotherapy after their mastectomy. The choice of the two treatments is usually by chance (randomization, page 321) and the groups are as large as possible to try to ensure that if there are differences in the rates of tumour recurrence or survival, this is due to the treatment and not a fortuitous finding. There are several large trials that have been underway for five or more years. They all show a benefit for younger patients receiving adjuvant chemotherapy. Even though this benefit is not *definitely* proven many would argue that if there is any potential advantage for adjuvant therapy it should be given to all young women who are node positive. This, however, ignores the penalty paid by those receiving chemotherapy (half of whom will never have recurrent cancer) – the definite side-effects of treatment. Early studies used simple tablets with relatively few side-effects but most specialists feel that combinations of drugs given by intravenous injection are more effective. Some trials of single drugs continue in Europe but nearly all adjuvant chemotherapy in the United States uses combinations of drugs. The side-effects (page 99) depend on the individual drugs being used but the following are common:

(a) Nausea and possibly vomiting for some hours after treatment.
(b) Tiredness and malaise.

(c) Partial or complete hair loss (very dependent on the individual drugs used).
(d) Susceptibility to infections, bruising, or bleeding.
(e) The emotional stress of prolonged drug treatment after the operation.

Treatment programmes vary, but the drugs are often given every 2 to 3 weeks for between 6 to 12 months. Appendix A outlines the common side-effects of single drugs so that an approximate idea of the effects of a particular combination can be gained from looking up the drugs to be used.

All women with cancer in lymph nodes at mastectomy should have the opportunity to discuss adjuvant treatment with their doctors. The options are: (a) no further treatment after mastectomy, (b) adjuvant chemotherapy using a drug combination, or (c) in some centres simple adjuvant therapy using one drug. In the United States combination therapy is recommended for nearly all patients; in Europe the position is more open and many doctors do not recommend adjuvant therapy or use simple adjuvant therapy.

There can be no clear-cut recommendation at present. The arguments for adjuvant treatment are strongest in young women but for older women (more than 70 years of age) there is little indication for such routine treatment.

Chemotherapy for recurrent cancer

Once breast cancer has relapsed cure is rare, but good contol of the disease of long periods can be gained. Patients who have recurrent or advanced cancer which is not responding to hormone treatment are often considered for chemotherapy (Chapter Fourteen). Many of the commonly used anticancer drugs are active in breast cancer. They are often used in a combination for best effect and will be given for at least two or three courses of treatment to test their effectiveness. A decision to continue treatment (if it is effective) or to change to an alternative treatment is then made and chemotherapy will often be continued for as long as there is evidence of a continued shrinkage of the cancer. Although many drugs are moderately effective it is rare for drug therapy to be curative though regression of cancer may occur for long periods. Unfortunately, chemotherapy is associated with side-effects and these are shown in Appendix A.

Patients with advanced or recurrent breast cancer can often live for many years with disease. They may require treatment intermittently (with hormones or chemotherapy) during this time but some patients (especially the elderly) have very slow growing tumours that require little or no treatment.

SUMMARY OF BREAST CANCER TREATMENT

Breast cancer is a very complicated disease. It is impossible to cover it adequately in one chapter and it is essential that patients discuss their treatment with experienced clinicians. Some guidelines can be given.

(1) All patients with a breast lump should see a doctor.

(2) A biopsy is always needed to make the diagnosis. All suspicious lumps should be biopsied, *most* are not cancer. The type of cancer operation should be discussed with the surgeon and if a limited operation is done it should be followed by radiotherapy.

(3) The behaviour of the tumour is influenced by the findings at operation. (a) the microscopic appearance may indicate a good outlook, (b) involvement of the lymph nodes under the arm indicates an increased risk of tumour recurrence, (c) the presence of hormone receptors suggests a high likelihood of response to hormone treatment.

(4) Radiotherapy after mastectomy is often used for cancers of the inner or medial part of the breast but its role in the treatment of cancers of the outer part of the breast is less clearly defined.

(5) Adjuvant chemotherapy is still controversial. A good case can be made for this treatment in young women (before or at menopause) with positive nodes. There is no case for adjuvant treatment in women over 70 years.

(6) Hormone therapy is usually the first treatment used if breast cancer recurs. Removal of the ovaries was the first treatment but drugs are now being used more frequently.

(7) Patients who respond to one form of hormonal treatment are likely to respond to other hormonal therapies.

(8) When tumour has recurred it is rare for cure to result from treatment and if the disease comes back after a response it is common to change to alternative treatments, either more hormones or chemotherapy.

(9) There are many active drugs in breast cancer; they are usually used in a combination.

(10) X-ray therapy is often very useful for controlling symptoms (especially pain) from recurrent cancer.

(11) Despite an inability to cure advanced breast cancer many patients survive long periods with or without treatment.

(12) Women with breast cancer need help to adjust to the situation. This help should come from family, the clinic, and if necessary from voluntary groups such as mastectomy associatons.

Notes

==================== GYNAECOLOGICAL ====================

Cancer of the ovary

Cancer of the ovary is less common than cancer of the uterus (womb) or cervix but causes more deaths. This is because it often does not cause symptoms until it is far advanced. The tumour tends to spread over the surface of the abdominal organs without invading deeply. No one knows what causes this cancer and and screening programmes to detect the tumour are of no use as the ovaries are so difficult to get at (Figure 36).

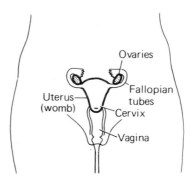

Figure 36 Diagrammatic representation of the female reproductive system showing the position of the ovaries

SYMPTOMS

Most patients present with vague symptoms and are found to have a tumour on examination. The common symptoms include:

- Abdominal discomfort or pain in the lower abdomen.
- Sudden swelling of the abdomen. This is due to the accumulation of fluid in a cyst or in the abdominal cavity (this is called ascites).
- Weight loss.
- Nausea.
- Occasionally shortness of breath due to accumulation of fluid in the chest (a pleural effusion).

DIAGNOSIS

A gynaecologist, will on pelvic examination have a good idea as to whether there is a tumour in the ovary. Further tests include:

- An abdominal and pelvic ultrasound (page 59).
- Chest x-ray.
- Blood tests.
- If ascites (fluid) is present then a small needle may be passed through the skin to suck some fluid into a syringe. This fluid is examined under the microscope to see if there are any cancer cells present.

TREATMENT

The outlook and type of treatment depends very much on the stage of the tumour (Chapter Ten). The extent of tumour spread is described by four stages:

Stage 1 — Cancer confined to one or both ovaries.
Stage 2 — Cancer has spread from the ovaries but is limited to the pelvic (or lower) part of the abdomen.
Stage 3 — Cancer has spread to the rest of the abdominal organs except the liver.
Stage 4 — Cancer has spread outside the abdomen or involves the liver.

The likelihood of response to treatment and outlook also depends on the appearance of the tumour under a microscope. Ovarian cancers are graded from 1 to 4 depending on their apearance; those which look most benign are grade 1 and those most malignant looking are grade 4. Because of the influence of *stage* and *grade* the treatment of the tumour is discussed using these factors.

Stage 1

When cancer is confined to the ovaries the chance for cure is high with surgery alone.

Surgery

(Chapter Twelve) The essence of surgery for this tumour is a careful assessment of tumour spread and then removal of all the

150

tumour and the local pelvic organs. If after very carefully examining the abdomen at laparotomy (an exploratory examination of the abdomen) the tumour is stage 1 then a good cancer operation includes removal of both ovaries, the fallopian tubes, and the uterus (Figure 35). The incision (cut) is usually made vertically over the lower abdomen as many surgeons do not feel that an adequate operation can be done using a bikini line incision (also known as a Pffanansteil incision). If such an operation is done the chance of cure is about 80 per cent. When the grade of the tumour is taken into account those with a good grade (1 or 2) have an even better chance of cure but those with a grade 3 or 4 tumour have less chance of cure and may be candidates for more treatment.

In young women who wish to retain their fertility the extent of surgery must be discussed very carefully. If a small tumour is confined to one ovary then there may be a role for less surgery in *selected* cases. The risks must be carefully balanced and fully discussed before operation. An incomplete operation increases the risk of relapse but retains fertility. If a lesser operation is contemplated then the other apparently normal ovary should be biopsied and examined by frozen section (a technique for immediate examination under a microscope) as involvement of both ovaries is common. If all the frozen sections biopsied are clear of tumour then an operation leaving one ovary, fallopian tube, and uterus can be performed. It must be stressed, however, that such a procedure should not be used routinely and is only appropriate in carefully selected cases where young women are anxious to have children and where the tumour is very small.

Radiation therapy

(Chapter Thirteen) No further treatment is required for those patients with a good grade (1 or 2) stage 1 tumour. For those with a poor grade (3 or 4) stage 1 tumour the chance of tumour recurrence is higher and some hospitals use radiotherapy. The best way of giving radiotherapy or chemotherapy for these patients is still unclear. In the past x-ray treatment was only given to the lower abdomen (pelvis) and tumour relapses occurred in the upper abdomen. For this reason many modern radiotherapy centres give radiation to the whole abdomen and pelvis. This treatment is very much more extensive but successfully stops tumour recurrence in the upper abdomen.

The first visit to radiotherapy is spent planning the individual treatment and patients should discuss the type of treatment to be given and its side-effects (Chapter Thirteen). Treatment is usually given for 4 or 5 days each week and if the pelvis alone is treated it takes 3–4 weeks. If the abdomen and pelvis are treated the time taken is between 6–8 weeks. Various special methods of treating the abdomen exist and these should be discussed with the patient.

The major side-effects are:

- Nausea and vomiting, especially when treating the abdomen.
- Loss of appetite.
- Tiredness.
- Diarrhoea especially when treating the lower abdomen or pelvis.

Chemotherapy

(Chapter Fourteen) Although a number of drugs are available for ovarian cancer they do not have an established role in treating early tumours. Some doctors are using anticancer drugs after surgery to try to improve the results — this treatment is experimental at present.

Stage 2

If it is possible to remove all evidence of tumour, survival is good. Tumour grade also reflects the likelihood of response and survival.

Surgery

The aim is removal of all tumour, both ovaries, fallopian tubes, and uterus (abbreviated to BSO and TAH). If this cannot be done as much tumour as possible is removed (known as debulking). Operations to preserve fertility have no role if the cancer involves other organs in the pelvis.

Radiotherapy

In patients who have had a complete removal of tumour, radiotherapy to the pelvis and abdomen (see stage 1) is used by some centres. If minimal tumour (this may not be visible) is left after operation (BSO and TAH) the chances of cure are high (60 per cent or more) when radiotherapy is used after surgery. When a complete operation is not possible and a greater bulk of tumour is left behind radiotherapy is less useful.

Chemotherapy

Chemotherapy is not used routinely in patients who have a complete operation (BSO and TAH) as radiotherapy is effective. In patients who have large amounts of tumour left after an operation for stage 2 ovarian cancer, chemotherapy is given in the same way as for patients with stage 3 or 4 cancer (see next section).

Stage 3 or 4

Unfortunately the chances of a cure in advanced ovarian cancer are not good (in the past less than 10 per cent of patients survived five years) but surgery remains important and the main aim is to remove as much cancer as possible.

Surgery

Even when cancer appears widely spread it is sometimes technically possible to remove all or nearly all visible cancer. This is because the tumour does not invade deeply into tissues and the cancer and organs to be removed can often be separated from the normal structures to be left behind. Ideally the operation should include removal of all tumour masses, the ovaries, fallopian tubes, uterus, and omentum (a large fatty sheet in the abdomen which is a common site of tumour spread). If this type of operation cannot be done then an attempt to remove as much tumour as possible is made. The least that should be done is to take a biopsy (sample of tissue) to confirm the diagnosis.

Radiation therapy

In stage 3 tumours when a complete operation has been done and there is minimal tumour remaining some hospitals use radio-therapy. This should be given to both the abdomen and pelvis (see treatment of stage 1) and results with selected patients in some centres have been encouraging. Radiation has no place in the treatment of patients who have a lot of tumour after operation or who have a stage 4 cancer.

Chemotherapy

For the past 20–30 years alkylating agents (see Chapter Fourteen and Appendix A) have been the first choice in the treatment of stage 3 or 4 ovarian cancer. About one-half of patients treated with these drugs have a useful response to treatment. Side-effects of these drugs, which are given by mouth, are usually few. The drugs may be given continuously or for several weeks each month. Cures with this treatment are very uncommon and the treatment is usually continued for several years or till the cancer relapses.

More recently drugs have been used in combination, *apparently* with better results. Such treatment is still being evaluated but of course produces many more side-effects.

The drugs commonly used (see Appendix A) are:

- Adriamycin.
- Cyclophosphamide.
- Chlorambucil.
- Cisplatin.
- Hexamethylmelamine.
- 5-Fluorouracil.
- Methotrexate.

A number of combinations of these drugs have been used but no ideal combination has been found. A rough idea of the side-effects of a particular combination can be gained from looking up the individual drugs in Appendix A. Combinations are more effective at reducing the size of a tumour but it is not clear whether long term remissions or cures are going to result. This type of chemotherapy is usually given intermittently (every 3 — 4 weeks) for a variable number of cycles (usually 6 or more) and if after several treatments the tumour is not responding the chemotherapy should be changed. At the end of the drug treatment if there is no evidence of tumour a second operation may be considered. At present second laparotomies (an exploratory operation) are being done more frequently but they are not yet of proven value. The *possible* advantages are: (a) they allow greater certainty in the decision to stop what may be unpleasant treatment if no tumour is found and (b) if tumour is discovered this may have become surgically removable and the operation can then be followed by more chemotherapy.

SUMMARY OF THE TREATMENT OF OVARIAN CANCER

(1) No predisposing cause is known and screening is of no use.
(2) Over half of all patients have advanced disease when first seen.
(3) Response to treatment and the chance of survival are related to the spread of the cancer (stage) and its appearance under the microscope (grade).
(4) Survival is good with surgery alone in stage 1 and further treatment is only indicated in patients with a poor grade tumour. Abdominal and pelvic radiotherapy may be given to these patients. Operations preserving fertility should be planned very carefully and are only appropriate in specially selected cases.
(5) Survival is moderately good in stage 2 disease. Surgery is the main stay of initial treatment. If a complete operation has been done abdominal and pelvic radiotherapy is given. If surgery is incomplete then chemotherapy is indicated.
(6) For stage 3 and 4 tumours surgery is still important and the aim is to remove as much tumour as possible. If a complete operation for stage 3 is done, radiotherapy to the abdomen and pelvis may be used. Other patients should receive chemotherapy. This may be simple treatment (an alkylating agent — Appendix A) which is moderately effective and has few side-effects. Alternatively a combination of drugs can be used, these cause more side-effects but are better in reducing the size of a tumour and *may* allow longer remission. These two types of treatment are being tested in

trials and patients should discuss the options with their doctor as no-one yet knows which is best.

(7) Second-look laparotomies are operations used to see if there is any remaining tumour at the end of treatment (usually chemotherapy). They are designed to: (a) allow the doctor to be as certain as possible that all the cancer has been destroyed before he or she stops treatment and (b) give a chance to remove any remaining tumour. No trials have tested if a second operation changes a patient's chance of survival and patients should discuss the advisability of a 'second-look' with their surgeon.

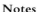

Notes

Cancer of the uterus (womb)

The lining of the uterus (Figure 37) is known as the endometrium and cancers of the uterus are often called endometrial cancers. The most common tumours of the uterus are not cancer at all, they are *benign* tumours called fibroids. These may cause excessive bleeding during menstrual periods (menorrhagia) or discomfort and a hysterectomy (surgical removal of the uterus) is sometimes done to prevent these symptoms. If fibroids are found no further treatment is needed as they are entirely harmless.

Cancers of the uterus usually develop later in life than fibroids. They are most common (Chapter Four) in women who are over-weight, have no children, have a late menopause, and have received long-term oestrogen drug therapy.

Screening programmes have not been useful. Although a Pap test (cervical smear, page 73) may pick up cancer of the uterus, it is not very helpful as it only tends to be positive in advanced cases.

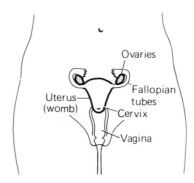

Figure 37 Diagrammatic representation of the female reproductive system showing the position of the uterus (womb)

SYMPTOMS

The most common symptom of cancer of the uterus is abnormal vaginal bleeding. This may be a change in periods if a woman is still menstruating and any woman with bleeding between periods should seek advice from her doctor. Similarly all women who have vaginal bleeding after their periods have stopped at the menopause should see their doctor. In most cases there is an innocent reason for the bleeding but the only way to be sure is to do a D and C.

Other symptoms may include abdominal discomfort or an offensive vaginal discharge.

DIAGNOSIS

A minor operation known as a D and C, where the lining of the womb is scraped away for examination, is the usual way of diagnosing this type of cancer (page 33). This operation is done for many different reasons and does not mean that cancer is present. Recently a new technique using an injection of a jet spray of fluid into the uterus has been introduced. It dislodges cells from the lining and these are collected and examined under a microscope. It is not available in some centres and a D and C is a more certain way of making the diagnosis.

If cancer is found the following tests are oten done before surgery.

- Chest x-ray.
- Intravenous pyelogram (IVP, page 48).
- Blood tests.
- Abdominal ultrasound (page 59) or CT scan (page 59).

TREATMENT

Surgical removal of the tumour is the usual treatment. Radio-therapy and hormonal therapy are also important.

Surgery

Before the operation begins the surgeon will carefully assess the extent of tumour spread. In addition to the tests above he will perform a careful pelvic (vaginal) examination under anaesthesia (known as an EUA). When the muscles are relaxed it is possible to get a much better idea of the size and spread of the cancer.

If the tumour is confined to the uterus and has not spread deeply into its muscular wall it is curable in about 90 per cent of cases by an operation removing the uterus and ovaries (a hysterectomy and bilateral salpingo-oophorectomy). An incision (cut) is made into the lower abdomen and patients should be up and about the day after the operation and are usually discharged after about 10 days. Full recovery from the operation may take several months.

If the cancer is deeply invading the muscular wall of the uterus then radiation therapy and surgery are often used together. The best treatment is probably radiotherapy given externally and internally with radiation implants (see Chapter Thirteen) and an operation to remove the uterus and fallopian tubes. Full discussion of the type of radiotherapy and the timing of surgery are important before treatment starts as each treatment is arranged for the individual patient. About half of the patients treated this way are cured.

Radiotherapy

When cancer has spread beyond the uterus and is involving the organs in the lower abdomen surgery has no part in treatment. Radiotherapy (given 4–5 times a week for about 4 weeks with or without radiation implants (page 91, Chapter Thirteen) is used and can provide good control of the cancer and its symptoms. The chance of cure is small (10 per cent), but is best in those with the least amount of cancer.

Hormonal therapy is used in patients with very advanced tumours or those who have recurrent tumour after surgery or radio-therapy. Progesterone, a female hormone, is helpful in about 30 per cent of cases and in those who respond the effect can last for a considerable time. The major side-effects of progesterone are occasional nausea and development of fluid retention (this may cause swelling of the ankles and legs, and if severe, shortness of breath).

Chemotherapy. Although there are some useful drugs available for this cancer only a few patients have a good response to treatment. Because of this drug therapy of cancer of the uterus is best reserved for patients being treated in trials.

SUMMARY OF TREATMENT OF CANCER IN THE UTERUS

(1) The use of long-term oestrogen therapy can increase the risk of this cancer.
(2) Early diagnosis is difficult and screening is of no use.
(3) Any woman with vaginal bleeding between periods or after the menopause should see her doctor immediately.
(4) A–D and C or jet washings are needed to make the diagnosis.
(5) In early cancers surgery cures nearly all cases.
(6) When the cancer is widely spread in the muscular wall of the uterus radiotherapy and surgery is necessary. About half of the patients will be cured.
(7) If the cancer has spread beyond the uterus few patients are cured and radiotherapy is used.
(8) Hormone therapy is very useful in about one-third of patients.
(9) Chemotherapy is only experimental.

Notes

Cancer of the cervix (neck of womb)

Cancer of the cervix (Figure 38) is the one tumour where screening to detect early cancer is routinely used and has a definite role. Despite this there is no general agreement as to when screening should start or how often it should be done. The subject is discussed more fully in Chapter Seven. Cervical cancer is most common in women who have sexual intercourse at an early age and with many men. Genital herpes (a virus infection which can be transmitted during intercourse) has been linked with cervical cancer though the evidence is becoming less strong. Cervical cancer is less common in women married to circumcised men.

Unfortunately those women at highest risk are also less likely to have routine screening pelvic examinations and Pap (cervical) smears (page 73). This is very important as the current management of cervical cancer is largely based on early diagnosis by smears. In addition to detecting cancer of the cervix, the Pap smear can recognize changes in cells (known as dysplastic cells) from the cervix which may develop into cancer (premalignant changes). Women with these changes should be watched very closely. Many do *not* go on to develop a cancer but some will.

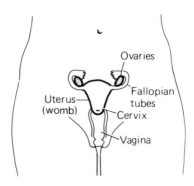

Figure 38 Diagrammatic representation of the female reproductive system showing the position of the cervix (neck of the womb)

SYMPTOMS

Ideally the diagnosis should be made by screening before symptoms appear, because by the time there are symptoms the tumour is usually far advanced. Symptoms include:

- Offensive vaginal discharge.
- Bleeding between periods or bleeding after sex.
- Late symptoms may include lower abdominal pain or difficulties in passing urine.

DIAGNOSIS

There is rarely difficulty in diagnosing this tumour as the cervix can be easily seen and felt during a pelvic examination and a sample of the surface of the cervix taken by a Pap smear.

If cancer is found the following tests may be done:

- Chest x-ray.
- Routine blood tests.
- Intravenous pyelogram (IVP, page 48).
- Pelvic ultrasound (page 59) or CT scan (page 59).
- Lymphanigiogram (page 51).
- An examination under anaesthesia (EUA) is carried out to estimate the extent of spread. This is done immediately before any operation, as the pelvic muscles are then relaxed.

TREATMENT

The management of cervical cancer in the early stages depends on the Pap smear findings and the stage (page 40). If cancer is suspected on the smear a biopsy is indicated. This may be at colposcopy (examination of the cervix using a magnifying instrument) or by a cone biopsy, where a ring of the surface of the cervix is removed.

Surgery

If on Pap smear and biopsy the tumour is confined to the surface of the cervix it is called an *in situ* cancer or stage 0. Ideally the treatment of a stage 0 cervical cancer is removal of the cervix and uterus (a hysterectomy) as this is curative in nearly all cases. In young women who wish to have children a cone biopsy only may be done and further surgery can be delayed till after she has had children, provided that *regular* check-ups do not show progression of the cancer. When her family is complete a hysterectomy should be done. Following a hysterectomy patients are up the next day and are ready to leave hospital at about 10 days though it takes 2–3 months to get back to normal. The incision (cut) is made over the lower abdomen.

- If the tumour has invaded the cervix itself it is referred to as a Stage 1 tumour. Either an operation or radiotherapy may be used to treat this stage and with both treatments most of the women will be cured. The main problem with surgery is the risk of complications. The commonest of these are wound and urinary infections or more seriously, although rare, are holes or fistules developing between the vagina and rectum. Treatment should be planned following discussion with a surgeon and a radiotherapist.
- When the cancer has spread beyond the cervix (stages 2–4; representing increasing spread) surgery plays no role and radiotherapy is the best treatment.

Radiotherapy

Radiotherapy can be used in stage 1 cervical cancer and is always used in patients with stage 2–4 cancer. The radiation is usually given by a combination of external and internal treatment (Chapter Thirteen), the radiation implants being placed in the uterus under anaesthesia. They are left in place for several days and then removed. The planning of radiotherapy is individualized and should be discussed with patients before treatment starts. Implants are used as they deliver a very high dose of radiotherapy to the area around the tumour.

Radiotherapy causes side-effects which include:

- Infertility and early menopause.
- Scarring and drying of the vagina that may interfere with intercourse.
- Diarrhoea during the treatment.
- Irritation of the bladder causing cystitis.
- Unusual late complications can include holes (fistulae) between the vagina, rectum, or bladder, and strictures (scarring and narrowing) in the rectum or bladder.

Chemotherapy

Chemotherapy is not very effective for this tumour and is not normally used except in trials testing new drugs.

SUMMARY OF THE TREATMENT OF CERVICAL CANCER

(1) Cancer of the cervix is more common in women who have had sexual intercourse at an early age and who have multiple partners.

(2) Pap smears are an established method of screening for this tumour and have played a part in reducing the number of deaths it causes. Women with abnormal (dysplastic) cells should have regular follow-up, but many will not develop cancer.

(3) A hysterectomy is standard treatment for stage 0 cancers and is curative in nearly all cases. In young women wanting children this may be delayed if there is careful planning of treatment and follow-up screening. Stage 1 tumours may be treated by surgery alone with cure rate of about 80 per cent.

(4) Radiotherapy may also be used for stage 1 tumours and is as effective as surgery; it is always used for stage 2–4 tumours. Cure rates depend on the degree of spread outside the cervix and vary from 1 in 10 to 1 in 2.

(5) Chemotherapy is experimental and not often recommended.

Notes

Cancer of the vulva

The vulva is the external part of the female reproductive tract. Cancers are relatively uncommon at this site and usually occur late in life. No causes are known.

SYMPTOMS

These are persistent irritation, pain, or bleeding from a sore or lump on the vulva. Women with these symptoms should see their doctor.

DIAGNOSIS

This is usually simple as the tumour is on the surface of the skin. A biopsy (removal of a small piece) is necessary to confirm the diagnosis.

TREATMENT

The usual treatment is surgical removal of the tumour and the cure rate is high, especially if the tumour is small. The surgical technique required depends on the extent of the tumour and in some cases removal of all the surface tissue of the vulva is required. Such an extensive operation takes a considerable time to heal and patients should discuss the details of the operation before treatment is started.

Notes

Cancer of the vagina

This is an unusual cancer that tends to occur in older women. In the past decade it has been seen in young women whose mothers were given oestrogens during pregnancy to try to avoid a miscarriage. Women whose mothers were known to have received hormones (usually stilboestrol) during pregnancy should have frequent screening examinations as early diagnosis is important.

SYMPTOMS

The usual symptoms are vaginal discharge or abnormal bleeding and pain.

TREATMENT

Surgery is not helpful. Radiotherapy with external and internal implant treatment (Chapter Thirteen) is usually required. The chances of cure are related to the degree of spread of the cancer. About one-third of all patients are cured.

Notes

Choriocarcinoma

This is a rare cancer of the placenta (afterbirth). The placenta is the organ that links a baby's blood circulation with that of its mother; it is important in supplying oxygen and nutrients. The tumour only develops in about one in every 40,000 pregnancies though it is more common in certain parts of the world, such as Malaysia.

About half of the cases of choriocarcinoma develop from an abnormality of the placenta called a hydatidiform mole. This is not a cancer itself and is uncommon (1 in 2000 pregnancies) but occasionally it may progress to a malignant tumour. All patients with a 'mole' should have very close follow-up to detect any change indicating cancer.

A choriocarcinoma may develop after a normal pregnancy or a miscarriage or abortion. One of the main characteristics of this tumour is its early invasion into blood vessels and very rapid spread through the body.

SYMPTOMS

These may be from a tumour in the uterus (womb) or from distant spread of the tumour.

- Continued vaginal bleeding after the birth.
- Abdominal pain.
- Cough caused by tumour spread to the lungs.
- Neurological symptoms because of spread to the brain.

DIAGNOSIS

This also includes an assessment of the local tumour and of any metastases. This tumour always produces a marker protein which can be measured in the blood. Human chorionic gonadotrophin, or HCG for short, is produced by the placenta during pregnancy and is also made by this tumour. It is useful for making the diagnosis and following the tumour's response to treatment.

TREATMENT

Although it is a tumour that spreads rapidly most cases can be *cured* by chemotherapy. Surgery and radiotherapy are usually not required.

This is a rare cancer and the treatment is very specialized and needs to be carefully planned according to the level of HCG in the blood. In most industrialized countries there are a few centres that specialize in the treatment of this tumour and **all** patients with this tumour should go to one of these centres. This is a curable tumour and the best chance for cure lies in expert treatment.

Methotrexate (Appendix A) has been the mainstay of treatment but other drugs are also used. Even when tumour has spread to the brain patients can be cured.

Notes

UROGENITAL

Kidney cancer

Kidney cancer, though relatively uncommon, is seen rather more often in men and usually occurs after the age of 50 years. Some of the chemicals used in industry can cause this tumour (Chapters 3 and 4) and smoking is known to increase the risk of kidney cancer by about five times. It is also called renal cell carcinoma or hypernephroma. The anatomy of the urinary system is shown in Figure 39.

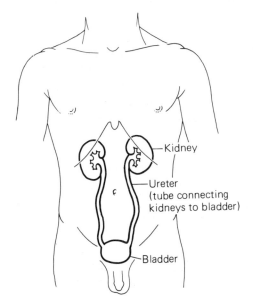

Figure 39 Diagrammatic representation of the urogenital system showing the position of the kidneys

SYMPTOMS

Often, these do not appear until the tumour is well advanced. The majority of patients develop symptoms because of local effects of the tumour, though some patients notice more a general illness first.

The common symptoms are:

- Blood in the urine.
- Pain in the flanks.
- Tiredness and a feeling of being 'one degree under'.
- Fevers.
- Weight loss and loss of appetite.
- Rarely, patients may develop symptoms caused by thickening of the blood. (The kidney tumour produces a hormone that tells the bone marrow to make too many red blood cells.)

DIAGNOSIS

Unless there are symptoms suggesting something wrong with a kidney, diagnosis of this cancer is sometimes tricky. On examination it may be possible to feel a lump in the region of the kidney and a sample of urine is examined to see if there are any signs of blood. If a tumour is suspected then further tests must be done and include:

- An intravenous pyelogram (page 48).
- Ultrasound of the abdomen (page 59) or a CT scan (page 59). If it seems likely that a tumour is present.
- An arteriogram (page 54) may be performed.

TREATMENT

Before treatment is decided on still further tests are needed to see if the tumour has spread. These include:

- CXR, whole lung tomograms (page 57) or CT scan of the chest (page 59)
- Venogram (page 54) to check whether the tumour is invading the main adbominal vein.
- Bone scan (page 62).
- Liver scan (page 63).

If these tests do not show any evidence of tumour spread there is a chance of a cure with an operation to remove the affected kidney (a nephrectomy)

Surgery

If a localized kidney cancer is removed patients have an excellent chance of cure. There is also a chance, though reduced, of complete cure in those patients who have involvement of draining lymph glands. In patients with widespread disease (metastases) a nephrectomy may be done if they are feeling well in themselves. Removal of the kidney is done to avoid local symptoms, but is not helpful in patients who are already ill because of spread of their cancer.

Radiation

This is being tested in trials and may be used with surgery though its use is unproven. It can be helpful if the disease has spread to bone.

Hormones

Occasionally patients have shrinkage of their tumour when treated with progesterone or androgen hormones. These treatments are relatively free of side-effects and are probably worth trying in advanced disease.

Chemotherapy

Drugs are unhelpful in the treatment of this tumour and should be avoided. There are no useful new drugs though trials of experimental chemotherapy drugs continue.

Although the treatment of metastatic disease is poor the outlook for patients with spread is uncertain. If patients are feeling unwell because of their tumour, survival is not good but some patients who have few general symptoms do quite well, despite continued metastatic disease. Very rarely this extensive disease may disappear; this is known as a 'spontaneous regression'. It is said to be more common if the kidney tumour is removed and has been used as a reason for operating on patients with widespread disease. Nephrectomy in this situation should only be done on those who are generally well and the main reason for the operation is to prevent local symptoms.

SUMMARY OF THE TREATMENT OF KIDNEY CANCER

(1) Certain chemicals are known to cause kidney cancer.
(2) Smoking increases the risk.
(3) Most patients develop local symptoms though about one-third only have general complaints.
(4) If the tumour is confined to the kidney most people are cured by its removal.
(5) Treatment for disease that has spread is poor though radiotherapy may be useful for bone spread. Chemotherapy should not be used. Hormonal therapy is relatively simple but is useful in only a few patients.
(6) Despite widespread metastatic disease the outlook is variable and occasionally patients survive years with cancer. Very rarely a spontaneous regression will occur.

Notes

Bladder cancer

This is the most common tumour of the urinary tract and usually occurs in people aged between 50 and 70 years. Aniline dye and other chemicals in industry (Chapter Three) may cause this tumour, and it is also more common in smokers. The anatomy of the urinary system is shown in Figure 40.

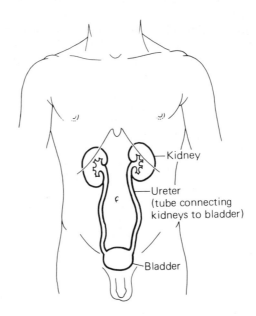

Figure 40 Diagrammatic representation of the urogenital system showing the position of the bladder

SYMPTOMS

- Blood in the urine is the first sign of cancer in threequarters of cases. It is worth remembering that most patients with blood in their urine, however, do not have cancer, though it

is a symptom which always needs investigation. The bleeding is often intermittent but this should not delay
investigation.
- Bladder irritability with frequency and pain on passing urine.
- In advanced cases lower abdominal pain may be a problem.

DIAGNOSIS

This should be relatively easy as it is possible to look directly into
the bladder using an instrument called a cystoscope. The tests used
include:

- Microscopic examination of the urine for evidence of blood
  or infection.
- Microscopic examination of the urine looking for cancer
  cells.
- Intravenous pyelogram (page 48), an x-ray outlining the
  urinary system.
- Cystoscopy is performed so that the doctor can look directly
  into the bladder and can remove (biopsy) any suspicious areas.
- Under anaesthetic a careful examination of the pelvis is often
  done as the muscles are relaxed.

If a cancer is found additional tests will include:

- Chest x-ray.
- Routine blood tests.
- Possibly, a liver ultrasound (page 59) and a bone scan (page
  62).
- Some patients may also have a lymphangiogram (page 51) to
  outline the lymph nodes.

TREATMENT

This depends on several factors. The stage of spread of the cancer,
its appearance under the microscope (grade – the higher the grade
the more aggressive its behaviour), and its location in the bladder.
The patient's general health must also be taken into account. This
tumour responds, up to a point, to both surgery and radiotherapy.

176

Surgery

Treatment depends on the stage and grade.

- Endoscopic resection of the tumour. This means the removal of tumour whilst looking through a tube into the bladder (cystoscopy). Under anaesthetic a tube is passed into the bladder through the urethra (tube from the bladder) and this allows the doctor to examine the surface of the bladder and to remove any cancer on the lining of the bladder wall. Patients with low grade cancers of the surface of the bladder lining are treated this way. Repeat cystoscopies are required and may be needed every few months, for years in some cases.
- Segmental resection of the bladder. This is an operation to remove part of the bladder containing a single large tumour. As bladder cancers are usually widespread this is rarely done, but if it is reserved for single large surface tumours of low grade it can be useful.
- Total cystectomy with urinary diversion. This is an operation to completely remove the bladder. As the bladder has been removed, the ureters (the tubes from the kidney to the bladder — Figure 40), have to be moved so that the urine can be collected. This is a difficult procedure and there are several ways that it can be approached. Before such an operation it is *essential* that patients discuss all the details and also see a stoma nurse (a nurse specially trained to look after patients undergoing such surgery). The operations are:

  (a) An ileal loop, which is perhaps the most common operation. The ureters are connected to part of the small bowel (the ileum) and this is brought up to the skin so that a bag can be used to collect the urine.
  (b) Rectal bladder. A colostomy (page 326) is performed so that faeces are collected in a bag. The ureters are then connected to the rectum which acts as the bladder.
  (c) Uretero-cutaneous. This means bringing the ureters directly up to the skin of the abdomen where a bag can be put over the stoma (the hole where the ureter is brought to the skin).

These types of operation sound quite mutilating but if used in carefully selected patients can be curative and work very well. Despite early anxieties most patients learn to adjust to having a urinary diversion and are able to lead normal lives. The operation is probably best reserved for patients with high grade tumours invading the wall of the bladder and some cases of lower grade surface tumours which are very unresponsive to lesser treatments. An operation for urinary diversion may also be performed in patients who have widespread disease with the intention of preventing a local problem.

Radiotherapy

Once again this is complicated and includes different techniques (external and internal implant therapy – page 91), for treatment at different stages of spread and combined treatment with surgery.
    Radiotherapy may be used in the following situations.

- After removal of low grade tumours of the surface of the bladder lining by cystoscopy has failed.
- When there are many large (wart-like), cancers of the bladder lining.
- When a superficial tumour changes to a high grade.
- As an alternative to removal of the bladder (cystectomy) when the patient's general health is poor.
- When simple treatment had failed to control high grade tumours that are in the bladder wall.
- Trials combining radiotherapy and surgery have been run for some years and continue.
- To provide control of symptoms such as pain or bleeding into the bladder when a tumour is widespread.

The technique of radiation is variable, but if implants (page 91) are not used then treatment is usually give for 4 or 5 days a week for 5–6 weeks. Side-effects of radiotherapy include:

(1) Discomfort and increased frequency of passing urine. These are temporary and can usually be controlled.
(2) Diarrhoea which can also be controlled.
(3) A risk of local infection.
(4) Late complications can include prolonged inflammation of the bladder, shrinking and scarring of the bladder, bleeding from the bladder, and prolonged diarrhoea.

If inplant treatment is to be used the technique will need to be discussed with the patient as the type of treatment may vary between patients.

Chemotherapy

Although several drugs are useful for bladder cancer there is no convincing evidence that combinations of drugs are much better than each drug used alone. The major drugs are adriamycin, 5-Fu, methotrexate, thio TEPA and cis platinum (Appendix A). All these drugs cause side-effects and this must be borne in mind when discussing treatment. About a quarter of patients will find these drugs effective but the benefits must be weighed against the toxicity and because of this there is no role for combination drug treatment except in trials. An idea of the side-effects of the drugs used can be gained from looking at Appendix A. Some drugs may be used by instilling them directly into the bladder though this remains experimental.

SUMMARY OF THE TREATMENT OF BLADDER CANCER

(1) Some chemicals are known to cause bladder cancer and smoking increases the risk.
(2) Care of this tumour is complicated and a collaborative approach (surgery, radiotherapy, and medical oncology) is often necessary.
(3) The amount of spread of a tumour and its appearance under a microscopy (grade) are important in choosing treatment.
(4) Surgery or radiotherapy may be used separately or together.
(5) The choice of the most appropriate treatment should be tailored for each patient and should be fully discussed before a final decision is made.
(6) If a cystectomy (removal of the bladder) is performed patients need a great deal of support and the advice of a stoma nurse.
(7) The chances of survival depend very much on the extent of spread and the tumour grade.

Notes

Cancer of the prostate

The prostate gland is located at the base of the bladder and is just in front of the rectum and can be felt during a rectal examination (page 32). Cancer of the prostate is common in older men and nine out of every ten cases occur after the age of sixty. The incidence increases with each year and 15 per cent or more of men over 60 years of age have the tumour but most are slow-growing cancers of low grade malignancy that never give trouble. No cause is known.

SYMPTOMS

Because it is commonly a slow-growing tumour many men die of other causes without ever realizing that they had the cancer. In others it is an incidental finding at an operation to remove a benign enlarged prostate gland (benign prostatic hyperplasia). Some tumours are found as a hard nodule in the prostate on routine rectal examination.

Most however cause difficulties in passing urine.

- Increased frequency of passing urine.
- Difficulty in emptying the bladder completely.
- Getting up at night to pass urine.
- Pain on passing urine.
- Blood in the urine.

Because the tumour tends to spread to bones patients may occasionally first notice pain in bones or pain from tumour in the pelvis (lower abdomen).

DIAGNOSIS

This tumour is diagnosed by rectal examination and then a needle biopsy (page 79). This is done under local anaesthetic, usually through the rectum and should not be painful. Because this tumour produces a chemical called acid phosphatase a blood test will be done to see if there are raised levels of the chemical in the patients blood.

Tests to look for spread of tumour will include:

- Isotope bone scan (page 62).
- X-rays of bones suspicious on the bone scan.
- Intravenous pyelogram (IVP, page 48).
- Lymphangiogram (page 51) to look at the abdominal lymph nodes.

TREATMENT

The choice of treatment depends on age, the extent of the disease and the patient's general condition. The options are surgical removal of the gland, radiation, or hormonal treatments.

Surgery (Chapter Twelve)

This is used in younger men, in good health, who have a cancer that has not spread beyond the prostate gland. Operations often affect sexual potency and radiotherapy may be used as an alternative treatment.

Radiotherapy (Chapter Thirteen)

When it is used in disease localized to the prostate about 50–70 per cent of patients will survive for 5 years and most will retain their sexual potency. Survival results with surgery are similar.

If the tumour has spread outside the prostate gland but is not involving bones then radiation is used. This may be together with limited surgery and implant radiation therapy (page 91) may be used as well as external radiation.

Hormone therapy

Growth of this cancer is affected by hormones and removal of male hormones and replacement with female hormones will slow down the tumour's growth. This may be done by removing the testicles (castration) or by giving female hormones (oestrogens) by mouth. Although these treatments sound drastic and affect sexual function they can give complete and prompt relief from bone pain or urinary obstruction that can last for several years. They cannot, however, cure the cancer.

182

Chemotherapy (Chapter Fourteen)

Chemotherapy should only be used in trials testing new treatments as the available drugs are of very limited value.

SUMMARY OF THE TREATMENT OF PROSTATE CANCER

(1) It is common in men over 60 years.
(2) It is often a slow-growing tumour.
(3) Symptoms of difficulty in passing urine are common.
(4) The chance of cure is best when the cancer has not spread beyond the prostate gland.
(5) Surgical removal of the gland usually causes loss of sexual potency but may be curative in the early stages.
(6) Radiotherapy may be as effective and does not affect sexual potency. Radiotherapy is also used for tumours that have spread locally.
(7) Hormone therapy is used for widespread disease. Chemotherapy is not routinely used.

Notes

Cancer of the testicle

Although they are relatively uncommon they are in fact the commonest type of cancer in young men (15–40 years). The only known predisposing factor is failure of a testicle to descend normally into the scrotum early in life (see page 19). There is no evidence that screening is useful but any lump in a testis should be examined by a specialist – a urologist. Although many men are reluctant to see their doctor with a lump in the testicle it is important to do so as this is one of the most curable tumours.

If a cancer is suspected a biopsy (using a needle or making an incision into the scrotum) should **not** be done. This may spread the cancer; an operation in the groin to take out and examine the affected testis should be done and if the testis contains cancer it should be completely removed. Men who only have one testis are perfectly normal sexually and can father children.

If the testis is shown, under a microscope, to contain cancer it may be one of two types.

- Seminoma.
- Teratoma.

Because the treatment of each type is different they will be discussed separately. The only common symptom of either type is a swelling (painful or painless) of a testicle. Occasionally swelling of one or both breasts may be noted.

SEMINOMA

This is commonest in the age group 30–40 years and is less 'malignant' than teratomas. They account for about half of the malignant tumours of the testis and spread from the testis to the lymph nodes in the abdomen. Occasionally it may spread further into the lymph nodes in the chest or even into the lungs.

Because of this, staging investigations (Chapters Nine–Eleven) are done to see how extensively the tumour has spread. These include:

- Chest x-ray.

- Lymphangiogram (to look at the lymph nodes in the abdomen).
- CT scan (in some centres) to examine the abdomen and chest.
- Blood tests to look for the marker proteins HCG and AFP. These proteins are only normally produced by teratomas so that if they are present in abnormal quantities this suggests that the tumour contains a mixture of seminoma and teratoma. Such tumours should be treated as a teratoma.

Staging

Tumours are divided into three stages as follows:

I   A tumour confined to the testis with no evidence of spread.

II A tumour that has spread to the lymph nodes in the abdomen.

III A tumour that has spread further and involves lymph nodes in the chest, the lungs, or liver.

Treatment

A combination of two or more types of treatment may be needed.

Surgery (Chapter Twelve)

An operation (using an incision or cut in the groin) is performed to completely remove the abnormal testis.

Radiotherapy (Chapter Thirteen)

If the tumour is stage I or II (as the great majority are) it is usual to give a course of radiotherapy to the lymph nodes in the abdomen. This will take about 3 weeks (treatment being given 4–5 times a week) and should not cause many side-effects though patients may notice some tiredness, nausea, or diarrhoea.

The vast majority of patients (95 per cent) are probably cured by this treatment.

Stage III

Extensive seminomas were also treated by radiotherapy in the past but chemotherapy is being used more commonly. The choice between these two types of treatment will depend on exactly where the tumour has spread to.

Chemotherapy (Chapter Fourteen)

Only a few patients have extensive disease or relapse after radiotherapy and are candidates for drug treatment. Recently chemotherapy of the same type given to patients with teratomas (page 187) has been used with good results.

MALIGNANT TERATOMA

This tumour spreads by the lymph system in much the same way as a seminoma but can also spread via the bloodstream. The risk of involvement of the lungs is therefore greater. Nearly all those tumours produce one or both of the proteins HCG or AFP. HCG, or human chorionic gonadotrophin, is produced by the placenta in a normal pregnancy and AFP (alpha feto protein) is also produced (by cells called yolk sac cells) in normal pregnancy. Some of the primitive or embryonic cells that produce HCG or AFP are usually present in a teratoma so that the protein can be measured in the patient's blood and this is very useful for monitoring the state of the disease at any time. The treatment, especially chemotherapy, of teratomas is complicated and they should preferably be cared for in a special cancer centre.

Investigations

These are designed to assess the extent of spread and will include some of the following.

- Blood tests for AFP and HCG.
- Chest x-ray.
- Whole lung tomograms (page 57) to look for small tumours.
- CT scan (page 59) to examine the abdomen and chest.
- Lymphangiogram (page 51) to look at the lymph nodes at the back of the abdomen.
- Blood tests to measure liver and bone marrow function.

Staging

There are a number of different staging systems in use so that this is a confusing area. However, the extent of spread divides roughly into three major areas.

I   Tumour is localized to the testis and all tests are normal including the markers HCG and AFP.

II   Tumour is involving lymph nodes in the abdomen.

III   In this case the tumour has spread into lymph nodes in the chest, into the lungs, or into the liver.

As important as the stage is the amount of disease, or bulk, at each involved site. The bigger a tumour the worse the outlook is.

Treatment

This will depend on the stage.

Surgery (Chapter Twelve)

All patients should have their testis removed through an incision in the groin. In the United States patients who, on investigation, are found to have stage I or II disease (unless it is very extensive stage II) usually have a further operation. This is to surgically remove all the lymph nodes at the back of the abdomen (a radical lymphadenectomy). Though this is a long and difficult procedure the patients are young and fit and tolerate it well. However, loss of normal ejaculation during sexual intercourse may result because of disturbance of some of the nerves at the back of the abdomen. The condition is known as retrograde ejaculation and usually means the man is infertile. In Europe and Britain radiotherapy is usually used instead of surgery. The results of treatment are excellent with surgery (95 per cent stage I and 85 per cent stage II are probably cured).

Radiotherapy (Chapter Thirteen)

In Europe patients with stage I or II disease are considered for radiotherapy. If there is involvement of abdominal lymph nodes only those with small tumours are treated. If patients are selected carefully the results are about the same as for surgery, but become less good if radiotherapy is given to patients with bulky teratomas. Radiotherapy does not cause retrograde ejaculation.

Chemotherapy (Chapter Fourteen)

Patients with extensive teratomas (bulky stage II or stage III) should be treated with chemotherapy. The most commonly used treatment is called the Einhorn regime after the doctor who originated it. It uses very high doses of three drugs, cis platinum, bleomycin, and vinblastine (Appendix A) and causes very many side-effects. Despite this it is very worthwhile treatment because the majority of patients can be cured. The major side-effects are:

- Tiredness.
- Nausea and vomiting with each treatment course.
- Abdominal pain after each treatment.
- Sore mouth.
- Risk of infection.
- Weight loss.
- Loss of hair.
- Pigmentation of the skin.
- Very occasionally damage to the lungs.
- Very occasionally damage to the kidneys.

Treatment is usually given over 5 days (in hospital) once every 3 weeks.

Other drug regimes using six or seven drugs are also being tested and may be as effective and are possibly less 'toxic'.

SUMMARY OF THE TREATMENT OF TESTICULAR TUMOURS

(1) Failure of the testicles to descend normally predisposes to a tumour.
(2) There are two major tumour types: (a) seminoma, (b) malignant teratoma.
(3) Testicular tumours should always be removed completely by an incision in the groin. Biopsies through the wall of the scrotum should not be done.

Seminoma

(4) They are commonest in the 30–40 age group.
(5) They spread by lymphatics.
(6) Most are localized to the testis or abdominal lymph nodes and can be cured (95 per cent) by radiotherapy.

(7) A few are more extensive and can be treated with chemotherapy or radiotherapy, depending on where they are. Most of these can be cured.

Teratoma

(8) These are most common in the 15–30 age group.

(9) They often produce a 'marker' protein – AFP or HCG.

(10) Their treatment is complicated and is best done in a special cancer centre.

(11) In the United States patients with stage I and stage II (unless it is a very bulky tumour) have a second operation to remove the lymph nodes at the back of the abdomen. The results are excellent (95 per cent stage I and 85 per cent stage II cured).

(12) Such an operation may affect ejaculation and fertility.

(13) In Britain and Europe radiotherapy is given to patients with stage I and to those with minimal stage II disease. The results of treatment are similar to those achieved with surgery (95 per cent stage I and 85 per cent stage II cured).

(14) Patients with more extensive disease are treated with chemotherapy. Although the treatment has many side-effects the results are excellent with up to 60 per cent of patients with advanced disease being cured.

Notes

RESPIRATORY SYSTEM

Lung

During this century lung cancer has increased in frequency more than any other tumour. There is no doubt that it is usually caused by cigarette smoking except in the case of one type, adeno-carcinoma of the lung (see below). The risk of cancer is related to the number of cigarettes smoked and when someone stops smoking their risk of cancer gradually falls, after about 10 years, to that of a non-smoker. Members of families who have several relatives with lung cancer may be at even greater risk if they smoke. Exposure to chemicals in industry (see Chapter Three) also causes some lung cancers though this is much less important than smoking. Screening tests have, unfortunately, not been successful.

Because the treatment of lung cancer is different for two main types, discussion in this chapter will be under two headings: (1) small cell lung cancer (oat cell), and (2) non-small cell lung cancer.

Small cell lung cancer (oat cell)

About a quarter of the cases of lung cancer are called small cell lung cancer. This is a rapidly growing cancer that quickly spreads to other parts of the body. Perhaps because of its rapid growth, it is the type of lung cancer that is most responsive to drug and radiation treatment. It is also known by the name 'Oat cell' lung cancer because its cells looks like small oat grains when seen through a microscope.

SYMPTOMS

Most patients, at first, have symptoms which are caused by the tumour in the lung though occasionally tumour which has spread elsewhere may cause the initial symptoms. The usual problems are:

- Cough with or without blood.
- Chest infection that does not get better with antibiotics.

- Hoarseness.
- Pain in the chest.
- Lump in the chest wall or above a collar bone.
- Swelling of the veins in the neck.
- Rarely, symptoms caused by tumour spread to the brain.
- Rarely, symptoms caused by the tumour making large amounts of hormones.

DIAGNOSIS

A chest x-ray will in nearly all patients, show a shadow which is suspicious of cancer. Although patients will be asked to cough up sputum to see if it contains cancer cells most patients will need a bronchoscopy (page 77). In this test, the surgeon is able to look into the air passages in the lungs (bronchi) and can take a piece of tissue (a biopsy) from any possible tumour. If a lymph gland (usually it is in the neck) is enlarged this may also be biopsied.

If it is not possible to make the diagnosis this way it is occasionally necessary for a surgeon to make a small cut (incision) just above the breast bone at the base of the neck. He will then be able to use a tube to look into the chest and to biopsy any odd-looking glands; this test is known as a mediastinoscopy. These tests are used to diagnose the cancer and further tests are then needed to see if the tumour has spread. These tests will include some or all of the following:

- Bone scan (page 62) and possibly x-rays of some bones.
- Liver ultrasound (page 59) or scan (page 63).
- CT scan of the chest and abdomen.
- Bone marrow aspirate and biopsy (page 66).
- Occasionally a CT scan of the brain (page 59) or brain scan (page 65)

TREATMENT

Small cell lung cancer is a very rapidly growing tumour which is nearly always widely spread through the body by the time the diagnosis is made. Because of this, surgery to remove part of a whole lung is rarely curative. The one exception to this is the occasional patient who has a simple lump or tumour in the lung, which is well away from the heart, blood vessels, and glands in the centre of the chest. In these patients the diagnosis of small cell lung cancer is often only made when the lump is removed and about one-third of these patients are cured by the operation.

An operation is not useful in other patients and treatment is by chemotherapy and radiation.

Surgery (Chapter Twleve)

Should be reserved for single tumour away from the centre of the chest and additional chemotherapy should be given after the operation. Patients undergoing chest surgery will have drainage tubes left in for several days after the operation but most will be up the day after the operation and are usually fit for discharge in about 2 weeks.

Radiotherapy (Chapter Thirteen)

Radiation treatment suffers from the same disadvantages as surgery – it only treats the cancer in the local area the radiation is aimed at. Although it was originally used to try to prevent symptoms due to tumour growing in the chest it is now mainly used together with chemotherapy or to treat symptoms.

Chemotherapy (Chapter Fourteen)

Treatment is given according to the extent of spread of the tumour. If the cancer is confined to one part of the chest only it is called a 'localized' tumour and if it has spread to any other part of the body it is called 'extensive'.

In each case the first treatment is chemotherapy and several drugs will be given in a combination, usually at 3-week intervals. A number of different combinations of drugs are commonly used and it is important to discuss the details of the particular treatment before it starts. The most frequently used drugs are:

- Adriamycin
- Cyclophosphamide
- Vincristine
- VP16–213

The side-effects of these drugs are shown in Appendix A and a rough idea of the side-effects of a combination can be gained from looking up each of the drugs.

Localized disease

As well as chemotherapy these patients are often given radiotherapy. This may be started together with the drug treatment or
may be delayed for several months while chemotherapy is given.
Neither approach is proven to be better though there are more
side-effects when the radiotherapy and chemotherapy are given
together.

The radiotherapy is usually given to the tumour in the chest 4 to
5 days per week for 3 or 4 weeks. Side-effects include:

- Tiredness and lethargy, this is made worse by the
  chemotherapy.
- Soreness on swallowing which is worse if the drug
  adriamycin is being used.
- Mild nausea.

Radiotherapy is often given to the head to prevent spread of the
tumour to the brain (see below). This will cause temporary loss of
hair, if drug treatment has not already done so, and can occasionally cause poor memory and loss of concentration for a couple of
months.

Depending on the way the treatment programme is designed it
may stop at this point or more chemotherapy may be given. The
usual period of treatment is about 1 year in all, though doctors are
unsure of the best duration of therapy.

Extensive disease

The only role of radiotherapy in widespread disease is to treat
symptoms and the most important treatment is chemotherapy.
Most patients respond quickly to drug treatment and if a patient
has had no useful response to drugs after two or three treatments
then it is doubtful that they will benefit from more chemotherapy.
If patients are responding then treatment is continued with the
intention of getting rid of all signs of tumour (complete remission,
page 288). Treatment is continued for about a year provided the
cancer is under control.

Brain radiotherapy

There is, unfortunately, a high risk of spread of the cancer to the
brain. Because of this it is common to give radiotherapy to the

brain as part of the treatment. Radiotherapy is given 4–5 times a week for about 2 weeks and is very successful in preventing symptoms due to spread to the brain. Many patients are very frightened by the thought of cancer in the brain or radiotherapy to the brain, but the brain is very resistant to radiotherapy and it successfully stops spread to the brain. Some doctors only give brain radiotherapy if the tumour is coming under control with chemotherapy.

Outlook in small cell lung cancer

This has changed in the last ten years. It used to be one of the most devastating cancers but is now very responsive to treatment. Most patients with localized disease have complete disappearance of the tumour with treatment and up to one in five of these patients *may* be cured and the rest have very useful prolongation of life. For those with extensive disease the outlook is not so good. Less than half will have a complete remission and very few will be cured. However, chemotherapy is useful for prolonging life in many patients. In the unlucky few who do not respond well to treatment, it is important to decide if it is useful to go on with further or different therapy.

NON-SMALL CELL LUNG CANCER

This is a collection of three different types of lung cancer which behave rather similarly. The names of these types are:

(1) Squamous or epidermoid cancer.
(2) Adenocarcinoma.
(3) Large cell cancer.

They are included together because their pattern of treatment is different from small cell lung cancer.

They do not grow as quickly as small cell cancer and because of this are less often widespread at diagnosis.

SYMPTOMS

These are usually due to the tumour in the chest.
- Cough with or without blood.
- Chest infection that does not get better despite antibiotics.

- Hoarseness.
- Lump in the chest wall or above a collar bone.
- Swelling of the veins of the neck.
- Rarely, symptoms caused by too much calcium in the blood.

DIAGNOSIS

The same tests are used as in small cell lung cancer (page 191) though fewer tests are done to see if the tumour has spread. As surgery is the most important treatment every effort is made to see if a tumour is small enough to be removed and to make sure there is no spread.

TREATMENT

If this type of lung cancer can be completely removed by an operation then the patient stands a chance of being cured.

Surgery (Chapter Twelve)

The number of investigations before an operation varies from patient to patient but will include a bronchoscopy (page 77) and possibly a mediastinoscopy (a minor operation to look into the chest with a small telescope). Patients will also have lung function tests to see if their breathing can stand removal of some lung. If the tumour is apparently localized and surgically removable then the patient is checked to make sure there is no tumour spread elsewhere (page 191).

When all these tests are completed, unfortunately, fewer than half of patients have a small localized tumour that can be removed. These patients, if their general health is good, will have the tumour removed together with part (lobectomy) or whole (pneumonectomy) of the lung on that side. Provided they have not had chronic lung disease patients can carry on as normal despite having one lung removed.

Of those patients who have this type of operation about one in five is cured. The operation is usually done by a thoracic surgeon and patients will have drainage tubes in their chest for a few days after the operation. They will be up the day after surgery and will usually be ready to go home about 2 weeks later. Full recovery takes a couple of months.

Radiotherapy (Chapter Thirteen)

Patients who have a local tumour that cannot be removed and no other obvious spread of tumour may be treated with radiation. This type of treatment is best reserved for treating symptoms and is very useful in dealing with pain caused by spread of the tumour. The frequency and length of treatment will depend on the aim of treatment and should be discussed with the radiotherapist.

Chemotherapy (Chapter Fourteen)

Unfortunately there have been few improvements in the drug treatment of this type of lung cancer. Although some patients respond to treatment there is no evidence that the patients live much longer. For this reason chemotherapy should, preferably, only be used in trials.

SUMMARY OF THE TREATMENT OF LUNG CANCER
(1) Many cases are caused by smoking.
(2) Screening is not useful.
(3) There are two major groups (small cell lung cancer and non-small cell lung cancer).

Small cell lung cancer
(4) This tumour grows quickly and spreads rapidly.
(5) Surgery is only useful for very few patients.
(6) Chemotherapy is the most important treatment.
(7) Radiotherapy and chemotherapy are given to patients with cancer confined to one side of the chest (localized disease).
(8) Chemotherapy alone is used for more extensive spread.
(9) Irradiation may be given to the brain to prevent spread.
(10) Most patients with localized disease have a complete remission; about one in five *may* be cured with radiotherapy/chemotherapy.
(11) Fewer than half of the patients with extensive disease have a complete remission and virtually none are cured.

(12) Many of the patients not cured have useful prolongation of life with treatment.

Non-small cell lung cancer

(13) Surgery is the most important treatment.
(14) Every effort is made to see if a patient is curable with an operation.
(15) Less than half the patients have an operation and about one in five of those who do are cured.
(16) Radiotherapy may be useful in controlling symptoms of the cancer if it is not curable.
(17) Chemotherapy does cause some shrinkage of tumour but does not often improve survival.

Notes

Head and neck

This is a very complicated section as there are many different places a cancer can develop in this region and they often behave differently and need various treatments. The tumours most commonly occur in elderly patients (more than 60 years).

When a doctor talks about head and neck cancer he means tumours developing in the mouth, salivary glands, nose and air passages, the voice box (larynx), and throat. Because of the many types of cancer it is only possible to discuss treatment in general terms. These cancers are most common in those who smoke and drink heavily. Some patients may have a premalignant lesion in their mouth called leukoplakia which can turn into a cancer.

SYMPTOMS

This will of course depend on where the cancer is, but the common symptoms are.

- Nose and air passages: bloody discharge from nose, obstruction to breathing through the nose, pain in the teeth and face.
- Back of the nose (nasopharynx): difficulty breathing, lump in the neck, damage to nerves supplying parts of the head and neck.
- Mouth: swelling or ulcer that fails to heal, pain, lump in the neck.
- Back of mouth (oropharynx): Pain or difficulty on swallowing, difficulty breathing, lumps in the neck, pain in the ear.
- Voice box (larynx) and surrounding tissues: Hoarseness, difficulty on swallowing, difficulty breathing, lump in the neck.

DIAGNOSIS

This is usually relatively easy as most of this area can be looked at or felt directly. The doctor will need to have a very careful look around the mouth, back of the throat, and voice box. In order to look at the back of the mouth a mirror, like dentists use, is warmed up before being put in the mouth (to stop condensation). The patient is asked to put his tongue out as far as possible and the doctor will hold the tip with a piece of gauze. He will then put the small mirror into the patient's mouth and have a look around. If necessary some local anaesthetic may be used to stop any gagging. Although, many patients are apprehensive before the examination it is quickly over and if expertly done is not unpleasant.

If a tumour is seen, or if a tumour is suspected to be in a spot where it would not be visible, then an examination and biopsy may be done under anaesthetic. Further investigation is needed if a cancer is found. This may include some of the following, depending where the tumour is:

- Chest x-ray.
- X-ray of the neck.
- Tomograms (page 57).
- Barium swallow (page 44).
- CT scanning (page 59).
- Ultrasound (page 59).
- Routine blood tests.
- Rarely, arteriograms (page 54).

TREATMENT

Surgery (Chapter Twelve)

Surgery of the head and neck is very specialized and should only be done by experts in this field. Any operation must be discussed fully with a specialist and the following important questions answered.

- Why is the operation necessary?
- How is the operation done?
- Are there any visible scars afterwards?
- Does the operation affect breathing, swallowing, or talking?
- What are the chances of cure and the chances of any unpleasant side-effects?
- Is any other treatment available and, if so, how good is it?

Many operations on the head and neck are very worrying and are sometimes disfiguring. However, if patients are selected carefully there is no doubt that many are cured by operations.

Radiotherapy (Chapter Thirteen)

The type of radiotherapy that is given depends on the tumour. Implants (page 91) may be used though external irradiation is more common. Some radiotherapy is curative, such as in early laryngeal cancer, but much is reserved for treating symptoms. Recently radiotherapy and surgery have started to be used together. The radiation may be given before or after surgery and patients receiving treatment should discuss the plan before treatment is started.

Chemotherapy (Chapter Fourteen)

Although several drugs can shrink head and neck cancers (cause a partial regression – page 288) chemotherapy has yet to make much of an impact on treatment. It is being used in trials before surgery in an attempt to shrink a big tumour so that it can be removed. This approach is unproven and is best restricted to these trials. There is no good evidence that combinations of drugs are much better than one drug alone in the treatment of advanced cancer. Some of the drugs used may be toxic and it is important to balance this against any possible advantages in these elderly patients.

SUMMARY OF THE TREATMENT OF HEAD AND NECK CANCER

(1) This is a collection of very different tumours.
(2) They occur in an elderly age group and are more common in men.
(3) Tobacco and alcohol are the main causes.
(4) Surgery can be curative if a small tumour can be removed completely. Some operations can be disfiguring and before any surgery all the options should be discussed.
(5) Radiotherapy can cure certain tumours and is usually less disfiguring than surgery. It is more often used to control symptoms.
(6) Surgery and radiotherapy are sometimes used together.

(7) Chemotherapy has yet to find a role, but is sometimes given to shrink a tumour before surgery or to try to control advanced disease.

Notes

LYMPH NODES AND BLOOD

Hodgkin's disease

This is a cancer that starts in lymph glands. It is most common in young people and also in those over 50 years. In the past it was a difficult disease to treat because it was so relentless and patients wasted away and died after a year or two. It is now one of the recent success stories in cancer medicine. Despite this it is still a complicated disease and referral to a specialist centre is desirable.

SYMPTOMS

The commonest symptom is a painless swelling of a lymph node (gland). Lymph nodes are scattered throughout the body and are linked by fine lymph vessels (page 51). Their job is to filter out excess fluid and to remove bacteria or unwanted particles in the body; they also produce some of the lymphocytes (a type of white cell) that get into the blood. Lymph nodes are concentrated in certain sites; the neck, under the arms, in the chest around the heart, and along the main blood vessels in the abdomen. The commonest site of enlarged nodes in Hodgkin's disease is the neck, but it should be remembered that most people with swollen lymph nodes do not have cancer, most glands swell in response to an infection. If lymph node swelling persists for several weeks advice from a doctor is needed.

Some patients have other general symptoms which can include:

- Drenching sweats at night. These may be accompanied by shivering (known as rigors) and feelings of coldness and heat.
- Loss of appetite and tiredness.
- Loss of weight.
- Severe itching all over.
- Pain in swollen glands on drinking alcohol which is a puzzling but uncommon symptom.

DIAGNOSIS

If there is persistent lymph node enlargement a biopsy (removal of the gland or a piece of it – page 65) should be performed. This can often be done by a minor procedure as an out-patient though, this will depend on where the lump is.

It is important that a biopsy is done by an experienced surgeon as future treatment may depend on the adequacy of the biopsy. If a lymph node cancer is suspected the surgeon should discuss the case with a pathologist before the operation so that tissue for any special tests may be collected properly. The interpretation of different types of cancer in lymph nodes may be difficult and a pathologist (the doctor who examines the tissue under a microscope) may need to ask the opinion of a specialist in this field. Four subtypes of Hodgkin's disease are recognized by pathologists: (a) lymphocyte predominant, (b) nodular sclerosing, (c) mixed cellularity, and (d) lymphocyte depleted. Although it was important in the past, the chances of survival are not much different for each subtype when modern treatment is used.

STAGING (page 36)

If the diagnosis of Hodgkin's disease is confirmed then the next step is to try to find out the extent of spread of the disease.

It tends to spread from one group of lymph nodes to another and then eventually into the blood and liver. The following tests are used first of all:

- Chest x-ray and sometimes whole lung tomograms (page 57) are done to see if there is swelling of the lymph glands in the chest and to examine the lungs.
- A lymphangiogram (page 51) to outline lymph nodes in the abdomen.
- Some hospitals may also use an ultrasound (page 59) or CT scan (page 59) to examine the abdomen.
- Bone marrow biopsy (page 66) to see if the bone marrow is affected.
- Routine blood tests.

A special staging system (page 36) is used for Hodgkin's disease.

Patients are divided into four stages according to the following criteria:

Stage 1: One group of lymph nodes involved, anywhere in the body.

Stage 2: More than one group of lymph nodes involved, but only if they are on the same side of the diaphragm (the muscle that divides the abdomen from the chest).

Stage 3: More than one group of lymph nodes involved, but on both sides of the diaphragm.

Stage 4: Involvement of the lungs, liver, bones, or bone marrow.

Patients are also divided into two further categories according to whether they have important symptoms or not. Those without symptoms are called A and those with sweats and fever or appreciable weight loss are said to have B symptoms.

The typical patterns of disease and its staging are shown in Figure 41. Staging is important because the type of treatment and its chances of success are closely related to the stage at diagnosis.

When these investigations are completed patients are placed in the appropriate stage depending on the results. If a patient has disease falling into stage 1 or 2 or if they have stage 3 with no symptoms (3A) they should be considered for a special staging operation.

Because there is a risk of undetected Hodgkin's disease in the spleen, abdominal lymph nodes, and liver most specialists recommend surgical exploration of the abdomen (a laparotomy). During this operation the spleen is removed and biopsies taken from many lymph nodes and the liver. A large bone marrow biopsy is taken as well.

The importance of the laparotomy is to ensure that all sites of disease are known so that radiation therapy can be planned if the Hodgkin's disease only involves lymph nodes. The spleen is removed to ensure that it is normal (if it is involved the risk of liver or bone marrow disease is much higher) and to protect the kidney from radiation. If the spleen is left and radiotherapy is given, the spleen which overlies the left kidney must be irradiated and this may cause permanent damage.

A staging laparotomy should be done by an experienced surgeon as it requires special care in examining all the possible sites of spread. In young women the ovaries should also be moved behind the uterus (womb) so that any radiotherapy does not damage them. A vertical incision over the abdomen is used and patients (who are usually young and fit) should be up the following day and be ready to go home in about 10 days.

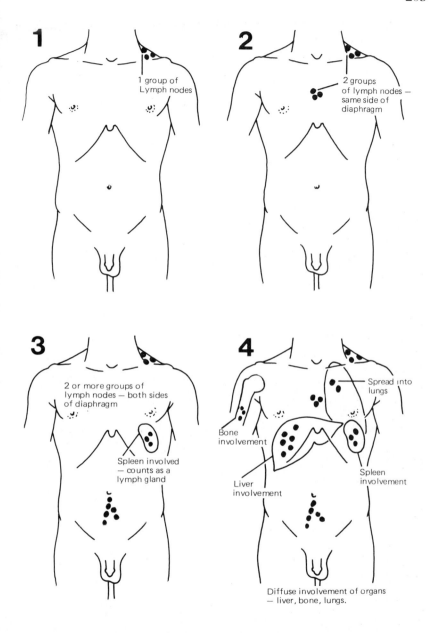

Figure 41 Schematic representation of the staging of Hodgkin's disease – see text for definition of stages

Removal of the spleen has few effects though children who have had a spleen removed have a higher risk of severe bacterial infections and some doctors give them long-term antibiotics or vaccines to try to prevent this. Severe infections are less of a problem in adults. Some doctors do not do a laparotomy or remove the spleen in children and the pattern of treatment is usually different from that of adults (page 284).

TREATMENT

This depends on the stage of the disease after careful staging investigations.

Stages 1A to 3A

Radiation therapy is the treatment of choice in those patients whose disease is apparently limited to lymph nodes. The chance of cure depends on the stage and is best in those with least disease (1A) and falls off as the amount of disease increases. The great majority of patients with stage 1A are cured with radiotherapy alone. Whilst just about half of stage 3A patients will have the tumour come back (relapse) after radiotherapy alone. However, most of those who relapse will obtain a second complete remission (page 288) with drug treatment. The cure rate is probably around 60–70 per cent for stage 3A.

Radiation is given to the involved lymph nodes and to all nearby lymph node areas. The overall extent of the radiotherapy depends on the amount of tumour spread. If the disease is above the diaphragm then the area or field to be treated is called a mantle (Figure 42(A)) and if the nodes are below the diaphragm a field known as an inverted Y is used (Figure 42(B)). When there is disease on both sides of the diaphragm and the patient has no symptoms (Stage 3A) the two fields are given and the treatment is referred to as total nodal irradiation (TNI). In the United States TNI is often used when the lymph nodes are only involved on one side of the diaphragm.

Radiation therapy (Chapter Thirteen) is carefully planned and then given for 4–5 days each week for 3–5 weeks. This is the time required to treat one field (a mantle or inverted Y). If total nodal irradiation is given then a similar period is needed for the second treatment: there is often a short gap between the two treatments.

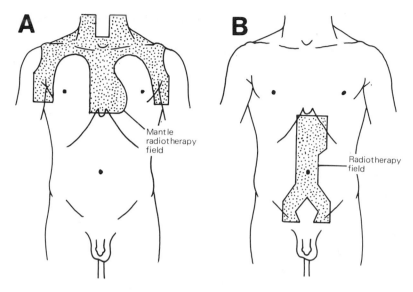

Figure 42 Schematic representation of the two common x-ray fields used for Hodgkin's disease: (a) mantle radiotherapy, (b) an inverted Y field. A radiotherapy field is the area to which the radiation is given

Side-effects vary from patient to patient and include:

- General tiredness that may take 1 to 2 months to return to normal if total nodal irradiation is given.
- Soreness on swallowing during mantle radiation.
- Nausea and occasionally vomiting, especially during inverted Y irradiation.
- Reddening and irritation of the skin at the site of radiation.
- Diarrhoea during inverted Y radiotherapy.
- Cough and irritation of the lungs after mantle radiotherapy.

All side-effects should be fully discussed with patients prior to treatment and if or when they occur. The radiotherapy should be given by an experienced radiotherapist as high doses are used over large fields and careful and accurate planning is needed to get the best chance of cure with minimal side-effects. Most patients tolerate this treatment well though radiotherapy in children has to be modified to avoid stopping bone growth (see Chapter Thirteen). Women who receive abdominal radiotherapy (an inverted Y) can be made sterile if the ovaries are treated. Because of this the ovaries should be moved behind the uterus (womb) at the time of staging laparotomy; this reduces the risk of infertility. In men the testes are not irradiated but should be shielded with lead during inverted Y irradiation.

Some trials using both radiotherapy and chemotherapy have been conducted to see if a combined approach is more effective. So far only very marginal advantages have been seen, and only after ten years. Because of the side-effects of this long and difficult combined treatment (see next section) it is not routinely used. Combined treatment may be beneficial in selected patients but we have still to learn which patients are best treated this way.

Stage 3B and 4

Radiotherapy is not used when the disease is advanced. Combinations of drugs are used for the treatment of stage 3B and 4, Hodgkin's disease (Figure 41).

There are several combinations that are commonly used. The first successful drug combination was known as MOPP and is the standard by which new treatments are judged. One of the reasons for looking for new drugs has been the side-effects of this combination. However, it is a very active treatment producing complete remissions in 70–80 per cent of cases and cure in about 40–50 per cent of patients with advanced disease.

The major side-effects (page 99) of MOPP are nausea and vomiting, pins and needles and sometimes weakness in the hands and feet, thinning of hair and suppression of the bone marrow. Other regimes appear equally effective but have not been used for as long a time. These drug regimes (all made up of the first letter of the drugs used) include MVPP, chlorambucil VPP, and ABVD. Discussion of the detailed side-effects is beyond the scope of this chapter and patients should always discuss the side-effects of chemotherapy before treatment. A rough idea of the potential toxicities can be gained from looking up the individual drugs of the particular combination in Appendix A.

The individual drugs in the combinations are:

MOPP – Nitrogen mustard, vincristine (also known as oncovin), prednisone, procarbazine.
Chlorambucil–VPP – Chlorambucil, vinblastine, prednisone, procarbazine.

MVPP – Nitrogen mustard, vinblastine, prednisone, pro-carbazine.
ABVD – Adriamycin, bleomycin, vinblastine, DTIC.

The drugs are usually injected into a vein and the treatment then repeated 1 week later. Tablets are taken with most combinations for 14 days after the first injection and there are rest periods of 2–4 weeks between treatments. Patients should ask for a detailed explanation of the timing (scheduling) of the drugs. If a regime that causes nausea and vomiting is used it is best to avoid driving home after treatment, though most patients do not need to be admitted into a hospital for treatment. A drip or IV infusion is set up and the drugs given by injection are injected into the fluid running into the drip. Following treatment the IV infusion is taken down and patients are able to go home. Antisickness injections or tablets are usually given at the same time.

HODGKIN'S DISEASE THAT HAS RELAPSED

Patients whose disease returns following radiotherapy do very well with combination chemotherapy used to treat advanced disease. For those patients who relapse after chemotherapy or who fail to respond to chemotherapy the outlook is not so good. Many will respond to further different combinations of drugs though the chance of long-term disease control is increasingly limited. In those patients who fail to have a complete remission with further combinations of drugs then control of the disease can often be achieved for long periods by using one anticancer drug at a time.

Such an approach is never curative but by changing the single drugs around according to the activity of the disease it is often possible to keep patients well for long periods. Some whose disease is resistant to treatment have lived with active Hodgkin's disease for ten or more years where this approach is skilfully employed.

LONG-TERM EFFECTS OF TREATMENT FOR HODGKIN'S DISEASE

There are two major long-term problems.

(1) Infertility (page 104). This is a major problem in men as nearly all those receiving MOPP, MVPP, or chlorambucil-

210

VPP combination chemotherapy are made sterile. It is claimed that ABVD (page 209) causes less sterility than the other combinations. Some women may become infertile or have an early menopause though this is less commonly a problem. Women having radiation therapy should have their ovaries moved behind their uterus at laparotomy in order to reduce the risk of infertility. The risk is greater in women older than 25 years who receive abdominal radiotherapy and chemotherapy.

(2) Second cancers. Unfortunately patients who are treated with both radiotherapy and chemotherapy are at an increased risk of developing leukaemia (page 219) or a non-Hodgkin's lymphoma (page 212). Though this risk is relatively small it is important if chemotherapy is being added to radiotherapy when the chances of cure with radiotherapy alone are high. ABVD chemotherapy is probably less likely to cause second cancers than the other types of chemotherapy.

Other long-term effects are uncommon and depend on the type of treatment given, they include scarring in the lungs and around the heart (radiotherapy), low blood counts (radiotherapy and chemotherapy), and an increased risk of severe infection after removal of the spleen.

SUMMARY OF TREATMENT OF HODGKIN'S DISEASE

(1) Hodgkin's disease is commonest in young adults; no causes are known.
(2) A biopsy of a lymph node must be taken to be sure of the diagnosis.
(3) Careful staging is necessary and may include a staging laparotomy. The presence or absence of symptoms is also important.
(4) Treatment is dictated by the extent of spread (stage).
(5) Radiotherapy is used for stages 1A to 3A. Some centres give chemotherapy and radiotherapy though this remains experimental.
(6) Chemotherapy using combinations of drugs, is given for patients with stage 3B and 4A and B disease.

(7) The results of treatment are good though the chance of cure is highest in those with the least extensive disease.
(8) Infertility is common in men treated with chemotherapy but is less of a problem in women.
(9) Leukaemia or non-Hodgkin's lymphoma can very occasionally follow treatment with chemotherapy and radiotherapy.

Notes

Non-Hodgkin's lymphomas

This group of cancers arises in lymph nodes and, although they are lumped together, they are a collection of tumours that often behave in very different ways. The conditions are separated from Hodgkin's disease (another lymph node cancer) and they can be recognized as being different microscopically and in their behaviour and response to treatment. Most non-Hodgkin's lymphomas occur in people over 50 years of age though some varieties are also seen in children. No cause is known.

SYMPTOMS

The commonest symptom is a painless swelling (usually in a lymph node) which may have been present for some time and which may fluctuate in size. Often lots of lymph nodes can be felt but, unlike Hodgkin's disease (page 202), disease outside the lymph nodes (*extra nodal disease*) is relatively common.

Other general symptoms that can occur include:

- Tiredness or a general feeling of illness.
- Loss of weight.
- Fevers or profuse sweating.
- Indigestion or abdominal pain if the lymph tissue in the stomach or bowel is involved.
- Pain in the left side and abdomen from an enlarged spleen.
- Lumps in the skin or itching if the lymph tissue in the skin is involved.

DIAGNOSIS

As with all cancers the diagnosis is made by taking a biopsy (removal of all or a piece of tumour). This can often be done as an out-patient procedure though it will depend on the site of the biopsy. Surgeons should ask their pathologist what specimens are needed if a lymphoma is suspected as special tests using fresh specimens are often used to determine the type of lymphoma (see below) a patient has.

When the diagnosis has been established the following tests are used to stage (page 36) the lymphoma.

(1) Chest x-ray.
(2) Lymphangiogram (page 51) to look for enlarged lymph nodes in the abdomen.
(3) An abdominal ultrasound (page 59) or a CT scan (page 59) may be used to examine the abdomen.
(4) Blood and urine tests.
(5) Bone marrow biopsy and aspirate (page 66).

A staging laparotomy (page 204) is not routinely used in the non-Hodgkin's lymphomas though, some intestinal lymphomas may only be diagnosed at an abdominal operation. The staging system used is the same one developed for Hodgkin's disease (page 203).

TYPES OF LYMPHOMA

Pathologists and doctors do not know enough about the non Hodgkin's lymphomas to allow agreement on a way of dividing lymphomas into various types. There are at present six or seven different classifications that try to do this. Although these classifications are based on different theories they all agree that non-Hodgkin's lymphomas can be divided into two broad categories. It is too complicated to discuss these classifications though the one most commonly used in the United States is named after its originator, Rappaport, and the most commonly used in Europe is named after the university (Kiel) that developed it.

Lymphomas can be divided broadly into two types.

Indolent lymphomas (also referred to as nodular lymphomas)

These lymphomas are often widespread at diagnosis (over half of all patients have involvement of the bone marrow). Most of them, when examined under a microscope, have what is described as a nodular pattern. They respond well to treatment with radiation or drugs but the disease is rarely eradicated. Even if treatment is not started straight away the outlook is quite good (most patients survive five or more years). During the course of the disease up to a quarter of patients will have a change of the lymphoma into an aggressive type.

Aggressive lymphomas (also known as diffuse lymphomas).

These are usually less widespread at diagnosis but grow more quickly and if left untreated are rapidly fatal. Some types respond well to treatment and there is a good chance of cure though this depends on the type of aggressive lymphoma and its stage at diagnosis. The chance of involvement of the tissues (meninges) around the brain is higher with some types of aggressive lymphomas.

Although the pattern of involvement (nodular or diffuse) in the tumour often corresponds with indolent or aggressive behaviour, there are exceptions and the pathologist can usually tell this by examining the type of cells in the tumour.

TREATMENT

Because of the different behaviour of the two categories of lymphoma their treatment will be described separately. Treatment also depends on the stage (page 203) before treatment.

(1) Indolent lymphomas

Stage 1

These are routinely treated with radiotherapy. The radiation field includes the known disease and nearby nodes and is not as extensive as that used for Hodgkin's disease (page 207). Unfortunately less than one in ten patients has stage 1 disease that may be cured by radiotherapy.

Stage 2–4

As these tumours are slow growing some doctors only treat patients with extensive disease if they are symptomatic or if the lymphoma is likely to damage an important part of the body. If this policy is followed some patients may not need treatment for long periods (up to ten years), though the number of patients needing treatment gradually increases with time. By about four years roughly half of the patients will have needed some treatment.

Both chemotherapy and radiotherapy are used and about threequarters of patients have a complete remission (page 288) with treatment. It makes little difference if the treatment is simple (local radiotherapy or a single drug) or complicated (combination chemotherapy – page 94, or chemotherapy and radiotherapy). It is therefore usually best to give a simple treatment with minimal side-effects unless a rapid shrinkage of tumour is required.

Though most patients have a complete remission the lymphoma usually comes back after a variable period (months to years). It is very unusual to get rid of the tumour completely and the idea of treatment is to keep the disease under control and the patient well. Survival is usually longer than seven years and patients may live for ten to twenty years.

Some patients have a change in the character of their lymphoma from a slow growing or indolent to an aggressive type. If this occurs they should be treated as for the aggressive lymphoma, and if they have not had previus drug treatment stand a reasonable chance of a complete remission and possible cure.

When chemotherapy is used for indolent lymphomas a single drug – often cyclophosphamide or chlorambucil (Appendix A) – is usually adequate. In some cases a combination of drugs may be used, the commonest of which is known as CVP (cyclophosphamide, vincristine, and prednisone). The period of treatment varies from patient to patient but is usually at least 6 months. The side-effects of treatment depend on the drug or drugs used and Appendix A can be used as a rough guide.

(2) Aggressive lymphomas

Stage 1 or 2

If after careful staging, the disease appears localized, radiotherapy is the best treatment. Two-thirds of patients with stage 1 disease and half of those with stage 2 can be cured. Some trials are currently testing the benefit of adding chemotherapy to the radiation. In certain types of aggressive lymphoma additional treatment is always given and patients should discuss their treatment programme bearing in mind the exact subtype of lymphoma they have. The radiotherapy fields are similar to those used for the indolent lymphomas.

216

Stage 3 and 4

Many aggressive lymphomas fall into this group and combination chemotherapy (Chapter Fourteen) is the best treatment. The chances of response to treatment depend on the particular type of lymphoma but over half of all patients will have a complete remission and nearly all patients will benefit from the treatment.

Several combinations are currently being used. The drugs in the common regimes are shown below and an idea of the side-effects of the combination can be gained by looking up the individual drugs in Appendix A. The toxicity and timing (scheduling) of each combination should be discussed fully before treatment is started. Most combinations are based on the same three or four drugs, they are the most active, and all are given intermittently (usually at 3-weekly intervals) for about 6 cycles.

CHOP – Cyclophosphamide, adriamycin (hydroxydaunorubicin), vincristine (oncovin), prednisone.
C–(M)OPP – Cyclophosphamide, vincristine (oncovin), prednisone, procarbazine.
BACOP – Bleomycin, adriamycin, cyclophosphamide, vincristine (oncovin), prednisone.
COMLA – Cyclophosphamide, vincristine (oncovin), methotrexate, leucovorin, cytosine arabinoside.
CVP – Cyclophosphamide, vincristine, prednisone.

Treatment is usually given for a fixed period of time and the need for further treatment then assessed. The period of treatment varies but is often six treatments though some doctors continue treatment for 2 cycles after a complete remission (page 288) has been attained. If the particular type of lymphoma is associated with brain involvement then radiotherapy to the brain and injections by a lumbar puncture (page 56) may be given as for patients with leukaemia (p. 280).

Side-effects of the chemotherapy vary from regime to regime and from person to person. The most common are:

- Tiredness and malaise – a general feeling of being unwell.
- Nausea and vomiting for some hours after each treatment.
- Loss of hair (this always happens with adriamycin, and it is also common with the other drugs).
- Risk of infection and bleeding due to low white cells and platelets (page 101).

- Tingling or weakness of the hands and feet. This takes some months to recover.

SUMMARY OF THE TREATMENT OF THE NON-HODGKIN'S LYMPHOMAS

(1) They are most common after the age of 50 years.
(2) There are many types of lymphoma which often behave in different fashions.
(3) There is no internationally accepted classification of the different types but all doctors agree on two broad types: (a) indolent lymphomas, (b) aggressive lymphomas.
(4) Treatment differs according to these two types and the spread of the disease. The same staging system is used as in Hodgkin's disease.
(5) Radiotherapy is used for stage 1 indolent lymphomas.
(6) Provided it is not causing symptoms or endangering the patient more extensive indolent lymphoma (stage 2–4) can be watched initially. Treatment is reserved for progressive disease causing symptoms and can often be delayed for some years. When treatment is needed it is best to give simple treatment wherever possible. Although this type of lymphoma responds well to treatment cure is rare.
(7) Long remissions can occur after treatment for indolent lymphomas but the disease nearly always returns.
(8) Radiotherapy is used for localized (stage 1 or 2) aggressive lymphomas and may be curative in many.
(9) More extensive aggressive lymphomas should be treated with combination chemotherapy. The chance for cure depends on the particular type and amount of spread. Involvement of the lining of the brain (meninges) is relatively common with certain types of aggressive lymphoma.
(10) If a patient with an aggressive lymphoma is going to have the disease return, this will usually happen within one year. Those surviving without relapse more than 2 years are probably cured.

Notes

Leukaemias

Leukaemia is a cancer which develops in the bone marrow. It can roughly be divided into two main types acute leukaemias and chronic leukaemias: this section only deals with the acute ones.

Although radiation and some drugs are known to cause acute leukaemia there is no obvious reason for the disease to develop in most patients and screening is of no use.

Most cases of acute leukaemia in adults are of a type known as acute non-lymphocytic leukaemia (also called acute myelogenous leukaemia, AML). Acute lymphocytic leukaemia, the type commonly seen in children, is seen in adults but is rare.

ACUTE NON-LYMPHOCYTIC LEUKAEMIA (ANLL or AML)

Acute non-lymphocytic leukaemia includes acute myelogenous leukaemia, myelomonocytic leukaemia, monocytic leukaemia, promyelocytic leukaemia, and erythroleukaemia as well as various subtypes according to the type of cell mainly involved.

SYMPTOMS

The symptoms of acute leukaemia are usually due to a lack of normally functioning cells in the bone marrow (page 101). About one-half of patients initially go to see the doctor because of a non-specific tiredness and other symptoms of anaemia. Others may develop infections (due to a lack of infection fighting white cells) that do not respond normally to antibiotics. Some may also have bruising of the skin, bleeding from the gums or nose, or bleeding into the urine or bowel caused by a lack of platelets needed for clotting.

DIAGNOSIS

This is usually easy to make. Any patient with symptoms suggestive of leukaemia should have a blood count. If leukaemia is present, the blood count will be abnormal with leukaemic cells (often called blasts) and reduced numbers of normal cells.

If the blood count looks like leukaemia the patient should be referred to a specialist (haematologist) who will perform a bone marrow test (page 66). This is a simple relatively painless test using a thin needle to suck marrow from a bone.

TREATMENT

Ten or more years ago there was no effective treatment for acute leukaemia and all patients died quickly. Nowadays drug treatment (chemotherapy) has greatly improved the patient's chances, though cure is rare.

Treatment is usually started soon after the diagnosis though it is worth getting control of any infection first. The greatest dangers from acute leukaemia are life threatening infections or bleeding and the patient will not improve until the disease is controlled and normal cells have returned to the blood. Because chemotherapy also reduces the number of normal cells in the blood it is common for patients to go through a prolonged period when they are very unwell and during this period they rely on the skill of their doctor to treat any infections or episodes of bleeding they may develop. Because of this need for expert support most patients are best treated in large hospitals or cancer centres.

Chemotherapy (Chapter Fourteen)

Chemotherapy is used in several phases, induction, consolidation, and maintenance.

Induction

This is the first phase of treatment using high doses of drugs in an attempt to obtain control of the disease. This is the most risky time during treatment as many patients are already sick and the treatment increases the risk of infection or bleeding. Nearly all patients will have some of these problems.

- Excessive tiredness or weakness.
- Nausea or vomiting after treatment.
- Fevers if infected.
- Sore mouth or thrush (page 100).

- Loss of appetite.
- Loss of weight.
- Temporary loss of hair.

Some patients do die during this phase of treatment but the alternative is nearly all the patients dying quickly if no treatment is given. Different regimes of drugs are used in different hospitals but the most commonly used drugs are (Appendix A): daunorubicin, cytosine arabinoside, and thioquanine. Several courses of treatment are usually needed to get the bone marrow back to normal (called a complete remission) and gaps between treatment will vary from 5 days to 14 days according to the blood count or bone marrow.

The whole of this phase is governed largely by the results of these tests so that the course of treatment cannot be predicted until their results are known. If the treatment successfully gets rid of the leukaemic cells the blood count will return to normal over the next couple of weeks. The patient will then rapidly start to feel better and the problems of infection and bleeding go away. Induction usually takes several weeks and most patients will be in hospital all or most of this time. About six to eight out of every ten patients will go into *complete remission* with induction therapy. This does not mean that they are cured only that the doctors can see no remaining evidence of the leukaemia.

Consolidation

Because it is likely that there are a few unseen leukaemia cells left in the bone marrow most patients receive several more treatments of high dose chemotherapy. This is known as consolidation and despite the high doses used it is usually much better tolerated by patients as their blood count is normal before they start treatment.

Maintenance chemotherapy

Even after consolidation therapy most patients whose bone marrow has gone back to normal (complete remission) will eventually have the disease return. In an attempt to delay this 'relapse' some doctors give their patients regular treatments of low doses of drugs. This treatment, known as maintenance therapy, is still being tested in trials and is not used by all specialists.

OUTLOOK

If treatment is not given most patients are dead within two to three months. Intensive chemotherapy produces a complete remission in 50–80 per cent of patients (this is partly dependent on age as older patients tolerate treatment less well). Those patients who do not go into a complete remission unfortunately, usually die quickly, often during their induction treatment. Patients in complete remission feel well and live longer (about 18 months on average) though a small proportion (less than 10 per cent) live for more than 5 years and may be cured.

The majority of patients who go into complete remission will relapse, though their life may be further prolonged with chemotherapy and a second or third complete remission is not uncommon. However, the chances of improved survival must be weighed against the very unpleasant side-effects of the treatment. Unfortunately if the intensity of the treatment is reduced the chances of a remission are much less. In young patients intensive treatment is nearly always worthwhile but the advantages and disadvantages must always be weighed carefully in older patients (more than 65 years of age) and less intensive treatment may be best.

Anyone receiving treatment for leukaemia needs a great deal of support and help from all those around them. Most feel unwell before treatment and at first are made worse by treatment. Even when the intensive first phase is over there is more hospital treatment, injections, and side-effects which are unavoidable and emotional support is of great importance.

ACUTE LYMPHOCYTIC LEUKAEMIA (ALL)

The treatment of this type of leukaemia is similar to that of widespread aggressive lymphomas (page 215).

Symptoms

These usually include:

- Enlarged lymph glands.
- Tiredness.
- Fevers and sweats.
- Bone pains.

- Symptoms from involvement of nerves, the spinal cord, or brain.
- Symptoms from an enlarged spleen.
- Symptoms from fluid or glands in the chest.

Diagnosis

This is made in much the same way as non-lymphocytic leukaemia and tests include:

- Blood count.
- Bone marrow.
- Lymph node biopsy.
- Chest x-rays.
- Isotope scans or x-rays.

Treatment

Several drugs are used together, usually given by injection, and treatment is given about once every 3 weeks. The most commonly used drugs (Appendix A) are:

- Adriamycin.
- Cyclophosphamide.
- Vincristine.
- Methotrexate.
- Bleomycin.
- Prednisolone.

A rough idea of the side-effects of any combination of these drugs can be gained from looking up the individual drugs in Appendix A. Most patients have much less in the way of side-effects than those with acute non-lymphocytic leukaemia as the blood count is usually less abnormal when treatment starts. Despite this, treatment is intense and there are life threatening risks from infection and bleeding.

Most patients go into a complete remission with treatment and during this period doctors usually recommend cranial prophylactic radiotherapy and chemotherapy (page 280) to try to prevent spread to the brain. This takes about 2 weeks and causes little toxicity.

Maintenance therapy is also used by some doctors in this type of leukaemia. Patients relapsing from a complete remission can be

224

put into a further remission with more chemotherapy though it is likely to last for a progressively shorter time with relapse. The leukaemia may also spread to the nervous system and this may become a difficult problem to treat. Injections of drugs (intrathecal injection – page 56) into the fluid around the brain and spinal cord are used and are usually given with radiotherapy. Unfortunately they are usually only of temporary benefit and the disease eventually returns in the nervous system or blood.

The chances of cure for acute lymphocytic leukaemia in adults is very much less than in children (page 278) and it is a much more resistant disease. However, more encouraging results have recently been reported in some hospitals and the treatment continues to improve.

SUMMARY OF THE TREATMENT OF ACUTE LEUKAEMIA IN ADULTS

(1) There are two major types: (a) the common acute non-lymphocytic leukaemia and (b) the rare acute lymphocytic leukaemia.

Acute non-lymphocytic leukaemia

(2) Some chemicals and irradiation can cause this leukaemia.
(3) Screening is not helpful.
(4) Patients are often very ill before treatment starts and most will die quickly without therapy.
(5) Intensive chemotherapy is used to treat the disease and this often makes patients more unwell and some die during this stage of treatment.
(6) Between 50 to 80 per cent of younger patients will obtain a complete remission. They feel well during this time though remission is usually temporary. A small number of patients have long remission (more than 5 years).
(7) After relapse some patients can obtain a further remission.
(8) The severe side-effects of the treatment must be weighed against the potential benefits – especially in the elderly.

Acute lymphocytic leukaemia in adults

(9) This is a much more resistant disease than in children.

(10) It is treated with combinations of several drugs.
(11) Side-effects are usually less than in acute non-lymphocytic leukaemia.
(12) There is a risk of nervous system involvement and cranial radiation and intrathecal drugs are often given to try to prevent this.
(13) Most patients go into a complete remission though this is usually temporary.

Notes

Chronic leukaemia

Chronic leukaemias can broadly be divided into two main types according to the type of cell involved: (a) myelocytes – chronic myloid leukaemia, (b) lymphocytes – chronic lymphatic leukaemia. Because the treatment and course is different they will be discussed separately.

CHRONIC MYELOID LEUKAEMIA (CML)

Another name for this condition is chronic granulocytic leukaemia (CGL) and the terms are interchangeable. The disease is common in middle age but can occur at any age group. No cause is known and screening is not helpful.

SYMPTOMS

These are often just a vague feeling of illness and include:

- Tiredness.
- Shortness of breath.
- Weight loss.
- Loss of appetite.
- Fevers and sweats.
- Pain in the abdomen from an enlarged spleen.
- Occasionally nose bleeds or bruising.

DIAGNOSIS

This is usually fairly easy. A blood count will show increased numbers of neutrophils (infection fighting white cells) and sometimes anaemia or a reduction in the number of platelets (clotting cells). Because this picture may be similar to that seen in the blood during an infection it is necessary to do a bone marrow test (page 66) to be certain of the diagnosis. Special chemical tests (leucocyte alkaline phosphatase) are used to help make the diagnosis and the chromosomes (carrying the genetic code) are examined. Nearly all patients with this type of leukaemia have a special abnormality of their chromosomes called a Philadelphia chromosome.

TREATMENT

Because many patients with this type of chronic leukaemia feel unwell they are usually given drug treatment. Unfortunately it is not possible to eradicate the leukaemia from the bone marrow and to cure patients. It is, however, possible to control the disease and to get rid of symptoms and return people to a normal life.

Chemotherapy (Chapter Fourteen)

As the treatment is palliative (to get rid of symptoms) a simple oral treatment is usually used. The most widely used drug is Busulphan (Appendix A). This is available in tablets of differing strength and it is given to patients until the white blood count falls to nearly normal levels. A reduced dose is then commonly used to try to keep the blood count near normal. It is important to have regular blood tests while on treatment so that the correct dose can be given. This treatment is usually remarkably well tolerated and many patients have their disease controlled for long periods. Other drugs can also be used with good results.

Surgery (Chapter Twelve)

Because the spleen of patients with CML can become painfully enlarged it is sometimes surgically removed. This can be very helpful in selected patients and is being tried out routinely in some trials.

Radiotherapy (Chapter Thirteen)

Radiotherapy may be used to treat the spleen and not only has an effect on the spleen itself but also reduces the white blood count and improves the bone marrow.

OUTLOOK

Although it is a chronic disease that is well controlled by simple therapy many patients eventually develop a more aggressive type of leukaemia (accelerated phase). This is usually very difficult to treat even when it is treated in the same way as acute myelogenous leukaemia. Despite this, about one in five patients in this 'accelerated phase' respond well to treatment. These patients can usually be picked out on blood and bone marrow tests as their abnormal cells look more like lymphocytes.

The outlook is therefore variable. Control of the disease and symptomatic improvement for a number of years is achieved in most patients but an aggressive and usually untreatable acute leukaemia eventually develops in most patients.

CHRONIC LYMPHOCYTIC LEUKAEMIA

This is a disease which produces less symptoms and a good proportion of patients are only found to have an abnormal blood count when they have a routine blood test, say before an operation. It is most common in the elderly but can occur at any age.

SYMPTOMS

This is variable but most patients only have relatively mild problems which may include:

- Generalized tiredness.
- Noticing swollen lymph glands which are usually painless.
- Fevers and sweats.
- Uncommonly anaemia, bruising, or bleeding.
- Recurrent infections.

DIAGNOSIS

This is usually simple as a blood count will show increased numbers of lymphocytes (a type of white cell). However, a bone marrow test (page 66) is needed to be sure of the diagnosis and sometimes a lymph node biopsy is done.

TREATMENT

This is an indolent disease that often requires no therapy for long periods. Because the aim of treatment is to control symptoms it is usually not given until the patient develops a definite problem.

This may include:

- Large lymph nodes pressing on important parts of the body (e.g. obstruction of a ureter–tube from kidney to bladder).
- Debilitating symptoms such as weight loss, fevers, and sweats.
- Anaemia or low platelets.
- Serious recurrent infections.

Cure is unfortunately not possible but good control of symptoms can be expected.

Chemotherapy (Chapter Fourteen)

The most commonly used drugs are chlorambucil and the steroid prednisone though any alkylating agent (Appendix A) can be used instead of chlorambucil. The treatment is usually given orally in low doses though high dose intermittent treatment may occasionally be given if a rapid response is required.

Radiotherapy (Chapter Thirteen)

This is rarely used as primary treatment but radiation to bulky troublesome nodes can be helpful in some cases.

This type of chronic leukaemia, unlike chronic granulocytic leukaemia, does not usually change into an acute form. However, it may with time become increasingly difficult to treat because the bone marrow is unable to work properly. This results in anaemia, a tendency to bleeding (low platelets), and a tendency to infection. These all make it difficult to give chemotherapy as it will make these problems worse, certainly in the short run.

OUTLOOK

This is a chronic disease and most patients will survive for five or more years even with no treatment.

Notes

Multiple myeloma

This is a cancer of the plasma cells in the bone marrow which is most common between the ages of 50 and 65 years. Plasma cells develop from lymphocytes and produce antibodies which fight infections. Because patients cannot make normal antibodies they are very susceptible to infections. The cause of myeloma is not known and screening is of no help.

SYMPTOMS

The disease usually involves bones all over the body though it may very occasionally be confined to one part of the body. The common symptoms are:

- Pain or discomfort in a bone.
- Recurrent infections that do not respond normally to antibiotics.
- Bones that break (fracture) after little or no injury.
- Shortness of breath.
- Undue tiredness.

DIAGNOSIS

This may be suspected on a routine blood count but special tests are needed to confine the diagnosis.

- Bone marrow (page 66) to look at the plasma cells.
- Blood test to examine blood proteins (plasma electrophoresis).
- X-rays of bones and sometimes a bone scan (page 62).

TREATMENT

Because the bone marrow is usually extensively involved drug treatment is needed. It is best to avoid staying in bed as this may make patients feel worse as the calcium in their blood may rise (page 304).

Chemotherapy (Chapter Fourteen)

The majority of patients will respond to simple treatment with tablets. The most commonly used drugs are melphalan (Appendix A) and the steroid prednisolone which are given once every 4 to 6 weeks. Occasionally several drugs given by injection may be used if the disease does not respond to melphalan treatment.

Most patients feel better and live longer because of treatment. This response often lasts several years.

Radiation (Chapter Thirteen)

Radiotherapy is very effective treatment for a pain confined to a bone. Most patients respond quickly and short courses of treatment will produce dramatic results with almost no side-effects.

OUTLOOK

Although myeloma responds to simple treatment it unfortunately usually escapes control after a variable period (years in most cases). It is then difficult to treat and most treatment should be designed to control specific symptoms.

The problems associated with uncontrolled disease are:

- Bone pain: usually well controlled by radiotherapy.
- Recurrent infections.
- Anaemia.
- Bruising or bleeding (low platelets).
- Generalized tiredness and weakness.
- Raised calcium in the blood.

Notes

234

===================== SKIN =====================

These are the commonest types of cancer and fortunately most are the curable. Because they are noticed early and do not spread quickly simple treatment is usually all that is needed.

Skin cancers are most often seen in fair skinned people who are exposed to a lot of sunlight. Ultraviolet rays cause skin cancer and screening clinics for malignant melanoma (see below) have been successfully used in Australia to cut the death rates for this dangerous cancer and other countries are starting similar programmes.

Rodent ulcers and squamous cancer

Both of these tumours grow slowly and only spread to other parts of the body late in their course. They remain localized for long periods but if they are neglected they will become incurable. Delayed treatment also means that more normal tissue must be removed with the cancer and this may be disfiguring, especially if it involves the face.

SYMPTOMS

A basal cell cancer usually develops in an area of skin exposed to sunlight and begins as a small firm and waxy protuberance that may ulcerate in the middle as it grows. The edges of the lump are often raised and it is said to look waxy or pearly.

Squamous cell cancers also grow on sun exposed areas. They often develop in precancerous skin lesions called solar (sun) or senile keratoses. At first it appears as a hard scaly lesion that as it enlarges breaks down in the centre and ulcerates and becomes covered by a scab. Only if the diagnosis of cancer is long delayed is it likely that symptoms of tumour spread will be present.

DIAGNOSIS

Anybody with a skin lesion that enlarges or ulcerates should go to their doctor though many of these do not turn out to be cancer. If it is cancer the chances of cure are good but are much better if the diagnosis is not delayed. Any suspicious lump should be biopsied and usually no further investigations are needed unless the lump is large or there is evidence of spread to nearby lymph nodes.

TREATMENT

The aim of treatment is removal of all the cancer with a margin of normal tissue. The way this is done will depend on where the cancer is and how large it is. The techniques available are:

Excisional surgery

This is the simple surgical cutting out of a lump. If the cancer is small the edges of the wound can be stitched together, but if it is large a skin graft is often needed. Most operations of this type can be done under a local anaesthetic.

Electrosurgery

This is the use of an electric needle that burns away the cancer. This is only used for small tumours and several treatments are often necessary. However, it can be done under a local anaesthetic and can be very useful in selected cases.

Cryosurgery

This is the use of liquid nitrogen to kill the cancer by freezing. It is usually reserved for premalignant lesions and very small cancers.

Radiotherapy

Radiation can be used to treat skin cancers but because treatment takes 3–4 weeks it is more troublesome. However, in certain situations such as tumours of the face it may avoid disfiguring surgery.

Tumours that have spread are more difficult to cure. The cancer usually spreads to the lymph nodes and an operation to remove the cancer and its draining lymph nodes may be done, an 'en bloc resection'. Radiotherapy may be of some use but chemotherapy is ineffective and toxic treatment should be avoided.

If a tumour is detected early the chance of cure is over 90 per cent but if the local lymph nodes are affected the cure rate falls to 50 per cent. Skin cancer that has spread to other parts of the body is rarely cured.

Notes

Malignant melanoma

Fortunately, this type of skin cancer is less common as it is much more malignant. It usually occurs in areas exposed to the sun but not always. The tumour develops in the pigmented cells in the skin and many start in moles or birthmarks. Although most people have moles the chances of one becoming cancerous are small and the routine removal of moles is not justified.

Symptoms

Any mole that changes must be examined by a doctor. Any of the following symptoms may be important.

- Irritation.
- Itching.
- Soreness.
- Change in size.
- Change in colour (darker or lighter).
- Bleeding.
- New moles around it.

Malignant melanomas often spread quickly and the key to cure is early diagnosis. If patients have any suspicious moles or pigmented lesions examination is essential.

Diagnosis and treatment

If a malignant melanoma is suspected then patients should be referred to a dermatologist or a surgeon. The suspected lesion should be completely removed and then examined under a microscope. Some surgeons may take a small margin of tissue with the mole but if it is shown to be a malignant melanoma they will need to do a further operation to remove a wide margin of normal tissue. Other surgeons, if they think it is malignant will take a wide margin of tissue at the first operation. In Australia special clinics have been set up to try to detect early cases. Anyone who is worried about a skin change can go to these clinics and this together with an increased public awareness of skin cancer has improved the cure rate for melanoma.

Surgery (Chapter Twelve)

Whichever approach is used a good operation must include the removal of the melanoma with a 2–4 cm margin of tissue around it and the resulting wound usually needs a skin graft to help healing. The chances of cure depend very much on how deeply the cancer has penetrated the skin.

There is still argument amongst surgeons whether it is a good thing to remove the nearby lymph nodes (page 81). This is only useful if the mole develops on a leg or arm as in other parts of the body the tumour can spread to different groups of lymph nodes. There are no definite guide-lines for when a lymph node resection should be done but if it is planned the operation should only be done by an experienced cancer surgeon.

Radiotherapy (Chapter Thirteen)

On the whole these cancers are not very responsive to radiation. However, if large fractions (big doses at each treatment) are given the tumours can be controlled. Radiotherapy is usually reserved for selected malignant melanomas of the face (where surgery would be disfiguring) and to treat some recurrent tumours. Repeated treatments are required over a couple of weeks but only about ten fractions are needed as the dose of each fraction is higher than usual.

Chemotherapy (Chapter Fourteen)

Unfortunately the drug treatment of this cancer is not very good. Several drugs can shrink tumours in about one in five patients but combinations of the drugs do not improve on this and, on the whole, toxic treatment should be avoided. The side-effects of the commonly used drugs can be found in Appendix A.

Immunotherapy

This is the use of various treatments to improve the immune system's ability to naturally destroy the tumour. Though some

240

types of immunotherapy can shrink the tumour if it is used directly on the cancer there is no good evidence that the chance of cure is improved.

The chances of cure of malignant melanoma are dependent on:

- Early diagnosis.
- The depth of penetration through the skin of the cancer.
- Good surgery.

Cure is unlikely if this cancer is shown to have spread. The tests that may be used to detect spread include:

- Chest x-ray.
- Liver ultrasound (page 59) or scan (page 66).
- Bone scan (page 62).
- Brain scan (page 65).

However, malignant melanoma is a strange cancer and widespread disease can, rarely, undergo spontaneous regression for years. Conversely other patients, apparently cured years ago, may have a tumour which suddenly recurs.

SUMMARY OF THE TREATMENT OF SKIN CANCER

(1) Fair-skinned people are more prone to develop skin cancer if their skin is exposed to sunlight.
(2) Any non-healing skin lesion or changing mole should be examined by a doctor — preferably a dermatologist.
(3) Basal cell and squamous skin cancers are just about the most curable of all tumours, but if diagnosis is delayed they can kill. Most patients are cured by a simple procedure to remove the cancer.
(4) Malignant melanoma develops in pigment cells and spreads rapidly.
(5) A wide excision of the melanoma is needed and this often means a skin graft. A specialist surgeon is often required.
(6) Radiotherapy is not usually used for treatment but can be helpful for recurrent lesions.
(7) Chemotherapy is not very useful and toxic treatment should be avoided.
(8) Immunotherapy remains unproven.
(9) The course of widespread melanoma is unpredictable.

241

Notes

CENTRAL NERVOUS SYSTEM

Brain

Most people are absolutely terrified about brain tumours. But in fact many tumours of the brain are not malignant. Those that are, may arise within the brain itself (a primary brain tumour) or grow elsewhere and then spread to the brain (a secondary brain tumour). Cancers of the lung, breast, and malignant melanomas as well as lymphomas and leukaemias are the tumours most prone to spread to the brain. Primary brain tumours, in contrast, rarely spread beyond the central nervous system (the brain and spinal cord).

The brain and spinal cord is surrounded by a protective bony case, the skull and spine. Neither of these allows much room for expansion so that tumours of the central nervous system quickly cause pressure symptoms as they expand.

PRIMARY BRAIN TUMOURS

The chances of cure depends very much on the type of tumour and exactly where it is. Tumours on the surface of the brain are more easily treated, whilst it is often too dangerous to remove deep tumours. This is because many deep structures in the brain are essential for life and cannot be operated on. Benign tumours are usually on the surface of the brain (the commonest is called a meningioma) but unfortunately many cancers are deep in the brain and invade surrounding tissue.

Symptoms

Brain tumours can cause symptoms either by affecting the area of the brain in which it is growing or by the increased pressure it causes within the skull. The symptoms caused by the local growth of the tumour vary according to which part of the brain is affected. Symptoms are therefore very varied and it is not possible to list the possible effects. One specific problem may, however, be seizures or epileptic fits. Seizures are caused by an area of irritation in the brain though it is worth remembering that most epileptics do not have cancer. Despite this all *adults* who develop epilepsy should have tests to rule out a tumour. The major symptoms of increased pressure within the skull (raised intracranial pressure) are headache, nausea and vomiting, and slowly increasing mental confusion.

Headaches

Everyone gets a headache from time to time and only very, very rarely is this due to a tumour so that it can usually be ignored. Severe persistent or increasing headaches should, however, be investigated and may be due to *many* causes, of which a brain tumour is only one.

Diagnosis

If a brain tumour is suspected then the patient should be examined by a neurologist who is a doctor specializing in the care and diagnosis of diseases of the central nervous system. A careful history of the problem and then physical examination often allows a skilled neurologist to piece together much of the situation. If he then feels there is a significant abnormality he may order the following tests.

- X-ray of the skull. Some tumours may show up as they contain calcium (as in bone) and others, although not visible, may push the structures of the brain to one side. Signs of increased pressure may also be seen.
- Electroencephalogram (EEG). This is a recording of the brain waves or electrical activity of the brain. During the test wires are tapped to various parts of the skull and the brain waves recorded from them. The test can only be interpreted by a trained neurologist, but may show an abnormal pattern of brain waves in the area of the brain where the cancer is growing. The test is simple and entirely safe.
- Brain scan (page 65). Brain tumours have a rich blood supply and the radioactivity that is injected accumulates in the cancer and shows up as an area of increased radioactivity (a hot spot) on the scan picture.
- CT scan (page 59). This technique is used to take very detailed pictures of the brain and can detect a small tumour and the excess fluid (oedema) that usually surrounds it. An injection of contrast dye may be given into an arm vein to highlight the cancer and this produces a temporary feeling of heat through-out the body.

- Arteriogram (page 54). If a tumour has shown up on the above tests an x-ray to outline the blood vessels within the tumour may be done. This not only shows up the exact location of the tumour but also reveals the blood vessels supplying it. This may be very useful to a neurosurgeon planning an operation. The technique of the test will depend on which artery is to be examined and patients should discuss the test before admission to hospital.
- Tests to exclude a secondary tumour. Before deciding if an operation is advisable it is important that a neurosurgeon considers whether the tumour is primary or secondary. Patients should be asked if they have had any other cancer and be routinely examined with particular attention being paid to the lungs (chest x-ray), skin (looking for malignant melanoma), the breasts, and then the urine is checked for any blood. If these tests are normal it is unlikely that the tumour has spread to the brain.

Treatment

This depends on the type of tumour and should always be done in a neurosurgical centre or a children's cancer centre.

Gliomas

These are the commonest brain cancer and are most often seen between the ages of 30 and 60 years, though they are also common in children. The important factors affecting the possibility of cure are:

- Site of the tumour. Some are easily removed but unfortunately most are deep in the brain and cannot be taken away completely.
- The appearance under a microscope. Some tumours do not look very abnormal (grade 1) whilst others may be very malignant looking (grade 4). Usually the higher the grade (1–4) the faster growing is the tumour and the worse the outlook.

The first treatment is medical. A steroid drug, dexamethasone (Decadron) is given by mouth to reduce any swelling in the brain. It does not shrink the tumour but decreases the fluid (oedema) around it. If the patient has had seizures antiepileptic drugs (phenobarbitone and/or phenytoin) are given.

Surgery (Chapter Twelve)

Surgery is then considered. Most of these tumours cannot be cured but some can if all the cancer can be taken away. It is not possible to fully describe such operations but an attempt to remove all or as much as possible of this tumour is often made. Before such an operation the hair must be shaved off (it will grow back normally afterwards) and then under an anaesthetic a flap of scalp is lifted up and a small section of the skull over the tumour is removed. The tumour and surrounding normal brain tissue is then removed and the piece of skull is then replaced and the scalp is stitched up.

One of the problems of brain surgery is the possibility of further damage caused by removing normal brain tissue from around the tumour. The likelihood of damage depends on where the tumour is and with some tumours the risk may be very small. There is often further swelling of the brain for a few days after an operation and this may cause increased symptoms but will improve over the next few days. Because of this, apparent increased brain damage after an operation should not always be regarded as permanent. As well as the usual improvement due to decreased fluid or oedema the brain can often adjust to damage and with intensive rehabilitation recovery from local brain damage may occur.

Radiotherapy (Chapter Thirteen)

Most patients who have had an operation for a glioma then have radiotherapy. Occasionally if a tumour is too deep-seated for an operation then radiotherapy may be used as the first treatment. Radiotherapy will slow tumour growth but rarely cures a brain tumour. The side-effects of the treatment are temporary hair loss and occasional mild nausea.

Chemotherapy (Chapter Fourteen)

Drug treatment remains experimental. A few drugs are active in these tumours and the most commonly used drugs are BCNU and CCNU (Appendix A) The effects of the drugs are modest but they do cause nausea and vomiting together with bone marrow damage so that the advantages and disadvantages of treatment must be discussed before it is started.

Outlook

Some patients with low grade tumours are cured whilst the others can live for years. If the tumour is of higher grade then the outlook is, unfortunately, poorer with few patients surviving two years, though occasional patients can be cured if the tumour can be completely removed.

Medulloblastoma

This is a tumour of young children which usually grows in the part of the brain concerned with coordination (the cerebellum) and because of this, a common symptom is incoordination. These tumours are fast growing and unlike other brain tumours, they spread to other parts of the brain and spinal cord. Despite its high degree of malignancy it is possible to cure this tumour.

Treatment should always be in a specialist centre and includes a combination of surgery, radiotherapy, and often chemotherapy. Surgery confirms the diagnosis and as much tumour as possible is removed. Following surgery radiotherapy is given both to the brain and to the whole of the spine. High doses of radiotherapy are given to the main tumour and this takes about 6 to 8 weeks. Lower doses are given to the rest of the central nervous system over 4 to 5 weeks. Chemotherapy drugs (Chapter Fourteen) are usually given into a vein by an injection or into the fluid around the spinal cord (an intrathecal injection into the CSF Page 280). It is obvious that the treatment of this type of brain tumour is highly complex and children should always go to a special cancer centre for treatment. Not only do they need expertise in arranging the best treatment, they and their family will also require special rehabilitation and support that is usually only available in such a centre.

One of the long-term effects of radiotherapy (Chapter Thirteen) is slowing normal bone growth. Because of this children who have radiotherapy to their spine as infants tend to be short and can develop curvature of the spine if care is not taken. Despite the complexity of the treatment and its side-effects over half of these children are alive after five years and more and more children are probably being cured. Parents must discuss all aspects of the treatment for this cancer before it is started as it requires a great commitment from everyone involved.

SECONDARY TUMOURS OF THE BRAIN

Spread of a tumour to the brain is more common than a tumour developing in the brain itself. The symptoms are similar to those of a primary brain tumour but additional symptoms may be caused by the primary tumour, wherever it is. Occasionally the first signs of cancer are symptoms from the secondary cancer in the brain but in most cases the patient is already known to have a cancer and then develops spread to the brain. Investigations will include:

- Skull x-ray.
- CT scan (page 59) or brain scan (page 65).
- Possibly an arteriogram (page 54) if surgery is contemplated.
- Investigation of the primary tumour.

Treatment depends on what is happening to the primary cancer but usually radiotherapy is given and this will control symptoms for months or even years. The main aim of treatment is not cure but control of symptoms, though if the primary cancer is controlled and tests show a single tumour in the brain then an operation to remove this may be attempted. If patients are selected carefully such an operation can be very useful, some patients living for extra years whilst some may be cured. However, surgical removal of a secondary tumour is generally not done if there is any other metastatic cancer as this will continue to grow.

OTHER BENIGN TUMOURS OF THE BRAIN

Benign or harmless tumours do not grow or behave like cancer but because they do cause pressure within the skull they need early treatment. They can usually be treated successfully by surgery or radiotherapy and never spread. The common tumours falling into this group include:

(1) Meningiomas (tumours of the lining over the brain).

(2) Pituitary tumours (the pituitary is a small gland at the base of the brain that controls the other glands in the body).
(3) Acoustic neuroma (a benign tumour of the nerve from the ear to the brain).

OTHER MALIGNANT TUMOURS OF THE BRAIN

There are a number of uncommon brain tumours but space does not allow discussion of their treatment. They include:

(1) Teratomas.
(2) Pineliomas.
(3) Neurolemmaomas and other rare tumours.

SUMMARY OF THE TREATMENT
OF BRAIN TUMOURS

(1) Brain tumours may arise in the brain itself (primary) or spread from another cancer (secondary).
(2) The skull and spine enclose the brain and spinal cord so that a tumour quickly causes symptoms of increased pressure.
(3) Symptoms are caused by the local effects of the tumour (this includes seizures) and by the raised pressure.
(4) The commonest primary tumours are gliomas. They are usually not curable though superficial low grade tumours can be cured by complete surgical removal. People with low grade tumours may live for years after partial surgical removal and radiotherapy but high grade tumours are usually rapidly fatal.
(5) Chemotherapy may be helpful to a few patients. More important drugs are dexamethasone (to reduce oedema) and antiepileptics to control seizures if they occur.
(6) Medulloblastoma is a very malignant brain tumour of children. Treatment is complex, including surgery, radiotherapy, and chemotherapy and should be given in a children's cancer centre. Despite its rapid growth and tendency to spread it is curable.
(7) Spread of cancers to the brain is probably more common than are primary brain tumours and their treatment is influenced by the state of the primary tumour. Usually radiotherapy is used to control symptoms but occasionally

an operation to completely remove a single brain metastases may cure a patient if the primary tumour is controlled.

(8) *Benign* tumours rapidly cause symptoms and should be treated as soon as possible. Surgery or radiotherapy can cure or control the disease for many years.

Notes

ENDOCRINE

Thyroid

The thyroid gland lies in the neck just below the larynx (voice box) and produces a hormone which, amongst other things, regulates the body's rate of metabolism. Swellings of the thyroid are common and most are not due to cancer. Anyone with a lump in their thyroid should consult their doctor to find out what the trouble is, but need not be too concerned about cancer as thyroid tumours are rare.

The only known cause of thyroid cancer is exposure to radiation. In the past, it was popular to irradiate the thymus (a gland in the chest) of children with all sorts of illnesses and it now appears that these children are more likely to develop thyroid cancer.

SYMPTOMS

Many thyroid cancers are found because of a simple swelling of the neck. There are different types of thyroid swelling and if it is diffuse throughout the gland it is unlikely to be a cancer. If only one part of the gland is enlarged it is called a nodule. This may be benign or malignant and may or may not produce thyroid hormone. If it does produce hormone it causes hyperthyroidism (over-active thyroid) the symptoms of which are:

- Nervousness.
- Intolerance of warm weather.
- Weight loss.
- Weakness.
- Rapid pulse or palpitations.
- Diarrhoea.

If the thyroid nodule produces hormone it is very unlikely to be malignant. Non-hormone producing nodules may be a simple cyst or may be cancer. Rare symptoms of advanced thyroid cancer induce hoarseness.

DIAGNOSIS

This is made by a combination of physical examination and a thyroid scan (page 64). A scan will show up an over active nodule as a hot spot and a non-functioning one as a cold spot. An ultrasound examination (page 59) may be done to see if a non-functioning nodule is a cyst or not. If a thyroid cancer is found it may be described, after examination under a microscope, as papillary (least malignant), follicular, or anaplastic (most malignant).

TREATMENT

Surgery (Chapter Twelve)

Thyroid cancer that remains localized to the gland itself can be cured by an operation to remove the thyroid (a thyroidectomy). The extent of the operation remains debatable and while some surgeons may leave some of the gland behind (a partial thyroid-ectomy) others will remove all of the gland and the neighbouring glands (a total thyroidectomy and excision of lymph nodes).

The problems of thyroid surgery include:

(1) Decrease or lack of thyroid hormone, leading to hypo-thyroidism (symptoms: slowness, intolerance of cold, thickening of skin, loss of hair, and constipation). Replacement thyroid tablets are needed for life and allow an entirely normal life style.

(2) Changes in balance of the body's calcium salts. Small glands, called parathyroid glands located in the thyroid may be inadvertently taken out or damaged during the opera-tion. If they are removed the blood calcium falls (hypo-parathyroidism) and this can cause muscular twitching, weakness, and seizures. Supplements of vitamin D and calcium will usually control the symptoms.

(3) Damage to the nerves to the larynx (voice box) may lead to permanent hoarseness.

Most patients do not suffer serious problems after thyroid-ectomy and for many it offers a high chance of cure. In patients with anaplastic cancers the tumour has nearly always spread early and an operation is not helpful.

Radiation therapy (Chapter Thirteen)

This is usually not used in the initial treatment of thyroid cancer but may be helpful in locally controlling anaplastic cancers.

Treatment of thyroid cancer that has spread (metastatic cancer)

Papillary and follicular cancers may take up iodine like a normal gland (this can be seen on a scan) and because of this they can be treated with radioactive iodine. In order to treat metastatic tumour a low dose of radioactive iodine is used to destroy the normal thyroid. No thyroid replacement is given and a high dose of radioactive iodine is then given monthly until the tumour no longer absorbs it. This is checked by repeating scans.

The radioactive iodine gives a localized but very high dose of radiation to the cancer. Although it rarely cures it can control the tumour for years and it must be remembered that the patient will need replacement thyroid hormone tablets for life.

Occasionally the growth of thyroid cancers is partly controlled by a hormone called thyroid stimulating hormone. Levels of this hormone can be reduced by giving high doses of thyroid hormone and this may cause some tumours to shrink.

Chemotherapy (drug treatment–Chapter Fourteen) is not very useful and only helps about one in five patients. The most commonly used drug is adriamycin (Appendix A) but toxic chemotherapy should be avoided.

OUTLOOK WITH THYROID CANCER

This is often a slow growing cancer and the chances of cure with surgery are good. Widespread disease can often be controlled for years though the outlook for those with an anaplastic cancer is unfortunately much worse.

SUMMARY OF THE TREATMENT OF THYROID CANCER

(1) Radiation of the neck may cause thyroid cancer many years later.
(2) Most cancers of the thyroid do not produce hormone.

(3) A thyroid scan will often show up the tumour.
(4) If the cancer is confined to the thyroid, removal of the gland gives a good chance of cure.
(5) Radiotherapy may be helpful in anaplastic cancers that usually spread rapidly.
(6) Radioactive iodine may be used to treat some tumours that will absorb the iodine.
(7) Drug therapy is rarely helpful.
(8) The chance of cure is best if the cancer has not spread outside the gland.

Notes

CANCER IN CHILDREN

The possibility of cancer in children is very worrying and frightens many parents, however cancer is rare and fortunately this is the group of cancers where we have learnt most and in which the chances of cure are highest.

A diagnosis of cancer in a child is a tragic event. But even advanced cancer in children can be cured and it is always worth trying treatment and aiming for cure. However, during this difficult time families need support from their own doctor and the team involved in the treatment. Because childhood cancer is uncommon, the treatment is complex and this emotional support is important, it is best that all cancers in children are treated at specialist centres. Only in a centre seeing a lot of children with cancer will there by the experienced staff who are needed for the best treatment.

If you have a child who has been diagnosed as having cancer they should be seen in a specialist centre, even if the treatment is then planned in conjunction with a local hospital. The chapters on surgery (page 79), radiotherapy (page 84), and drug therapy (page 93) all apply to children and there are doctors who specialize in using each of these treatments in children only.

Table 8 Relative frequency (per cent) of the common childhood cancers

Tumour type	Relative proportion (%)
Leukaemia	30
Lymphoma	8
Hodgkin's disease	6
Nervous system tumours	12
Bone sarcoma	12
Soft tissue sarcoma	12
Neuroblastoma	10
Wilm's (kidney)	8
Others	2

This section deals with the diagnosis and treatment of the common childhood tumours. The relative frequency of these cancers is shown in Table 8.

Doctors looking after childhood cancers have been in the forefront of new treatments for cancer and many children are treated in trials testing new treatments (Chapter twenty). Parents will need to discuss with their doctor the possible inclusion of their child in a trial.

During treatment many of these children are at great risk from ordinary childhood infections and parents should also talk to the doctors about the risks and what can be done to reduce this.

Neuroblastoma

About one in ten cases of childhood cancer is a neuroblastoma. The tumour grows from cells that form the tissue of special nerves called sympathetic nerves. Because these tissues are widespread the tumour can arise in many sites but most are at the back of the abdomen and nearly half are in an adrenal gland just above a kidney.

The cancer tends to spread locally by lymphatics (page 36) and by the blood so that it may be in various parts of the body at diagnosis. It is a cancer that is most common very early in life and half of all patients are younger than 2 years of age and fortunately the outlook is best in these very young children.

This tumour often produces substances (called catecholamines) that may be measured in the urine and these help in establishing the diagnosis and following its response to treatment. They may also cause an increase in blood pressure as they are similar to adrenalin. It should always be remembered that very young children (less than 1 year) have a very good chance of cure even if the tumour is widespread.

Symptoms

These may be caused by the local tumour or may be due to spread of the cancer. The commonest effects are:

- Swelling of the abdomen or a lump in the abdomen.
- Swelling in the neck.
- Prolonged jaundice after birth.
- Cough, shortness of breath.
- High blood pressure.
- Weight loss.
- Poor appetite.
- Protrusion of an eye (exophthalmos) caused by a tumour behind the eye.

Diagnosis and Staging

The aim of investigation is to confirm the diagnosis and then to see if there is any spread of the cancer. A biopsy is needed before treatment is finally planned but in many cases the diagnosis will be strongly suspected before this is done.

Routine investigations include some of the following tests:

- X-ray of chest and abdomen. About half of the tumours contain some calcium (like bone) which shows up on a plain x-ray. X-rays of bone may also show spread of the tumour and a bone survey may be done.
- IVP (page 48) This often shows that the kidney is pushed over by the tumour.
- 24 hours urine collection. About 8 in 10 patients will have extra amounts of catecholamines (one of which is called VMA) in their urine and this can be measured. Before a urine collection for these substances can be done it is important that the child is on a special diet. The following foods should **not** be eaten as they will affect the test, which is often called a VMA test.

  (1) Tea.
  (2) Coca Cola and other colas.
  (3) Chocolate.
  (4) Vanilla.
  (5) Bananas.
  (6) Grapes.
  (7) Oranges.
  (8) Tomatoes.
  (9) Aspirin.
(10) Sulphur antibiotics.
(11) Some cough mixtures.

- Arteriography (page 54). An arteriogram outlining the blood supply of the tumour is often useful.
- Lymphangiography (page 51) may be used to outline lymph nodes in the abdomen and is usually done under a general anaesthetic.
- Bone marrow aspirate (page 66) This is done under a general anaesthetic and may show spread to the bone marrow.

Treatment

Surgery (Chapter Twelve)

If a child does not have any spread of the tumour and the tumour can be totally removed there is a cure rate of about 90 per cent regardless of age. However, if only part of the tumour can be removed then it is probably better only to do a biopsy to confirm the diagnosis. Operations to remove part of this tumour are usually not helpful and following the biopsy it is best to just mark out the area of the cancer with some metal clips. These will show up on an x-ray and help with radiotherapy planning. Sometimes another operation may be considered after radiotherapy and chemo-therapy.

The nature of any operation depends on the size and site of the tumour but young children are very resilient and are able to stand up to major operations.

Radiotherapy (Chapter Thirteen)

Radiotherapy may be used to treat any tumour left behind after an incomplete operation or a tumour which could not be removed at all. The radiotherapy may be given with the intention of cure or for palliation (treatment of symptoms); this depends on the size of the cancer and where it is. If a surgeon has marked out the tumour with metal clips this helps in the treatment planning.

The tumour is usually quite sensitive to irradiation and low doses may be given; older children tend to have less sensitive tumours which need more irradiation.

The treatment is usually given over 3 to 4 weeks in small divided doses. Details of the treatment programme should be discussed fully before treatment as it needs to be tailored for the individual patient. Radiotherapy is usually well tolerated but needs care in planning as it can cause damage to bone growth.

Chemotherapy (Chapter Fourteen)

Drug therapy is usually given in a treatment programme including surgery and radiotherapy. Although tumours often respond to treatment the chances of a complete remission (page 288) and cure are not good if the tumour is very extensive.

Various combinations of drugs are used and an idea of the side-effects of a combination can be gathered by looking up the individual drugs in Appendix A. Although chemotherapy has many side-effects young children usually cope with these much better than adults.

CHANCES OF CURE

The chance of cure depends on several factors.

(1) Age. The younger a child is the greater are the chances of survival. For those children less than 1 year about eight of every ten are cured. After this age the chance of cure gradually diminishes.
(2) Stage. The degree of spread of neuroblastoma is broken down into four stages and the higher the stage the less is the chance for cure.

In the group of very young children (less than 1 year) spontaneous regressions are quite common. A special stage (IV–S) is used to pick out those young children who have widespread disease and who are likely to be cured with minimal treatment.

SUMMARY OF THE TREATMENT OF NEUROBLASTOMAS

(1) Most occur in the abdomen, usually around the adrenal gland, though they can grow in the chest or head and neck.
(2) Many of these tumours produce substances (catecholamines) that can be found in the urine. These can be used to help make the diagnosis and to follow the progress of the child.
(3) Surgery is used to make the diagnosis (biopsy) or if possible to completely remove the cancer.
(4) Radiotherapy is given for tumours that cannot be surgically taken away.
(5) Drug therapy is not very active but is often used together with surgery and radiotherapy.
(6) Despite the intensive treatment most children are able to tolerate this as they are more resilient than adults.
(7) The chance for cure is best in very young patients.

260

(8) A special stage (IVS) is used to describe the widespread disease in infants less than 1 year that may go away by itself (a spontaneous regression) and therefore needs little treatment.
(9) This cancer should be treated in a special centre.
(10) The whole family needs the support of their own doctor and the team treating the child.

Notes

Wilm's tumour

Wilm's tumour, also known as nephroblastoma, is one of the commonest cancers in children and usually occurs betweent he ages of one to five years. Although *most* children do not have any obvious genetic abnormality, Wilm's tumour is more common in children with the following unusual birth abnormalities:

(1) Abnormalities of the urogenital system (kidney, ureters, and bladder).
(2) Over-growth one half of the body (hemihypertrophy).
(3) Partial or complete absence of the iris in the eye.

SYMPTOMS

This cancer may cause several non-specific symptoms. There include abdominal discomfort, gastrointestinal upset, fever, and blood in the urine (haematuria). However, accidental discovery of a lump in the abdomen is often the first sign of the tumour. It is usually felt as a firm, irregular, and non-tender mass. In some children both kidneys may be affected.

DIAGNOSIS

If a Wilm's tumour is suspected a series of x-rays and scans (under general anaesthetic if required) may be used to try to confirm the diagnosis before any operation is contemplated. X-rays will include the following:

- A plain x-ray of the abdomen to see if a lump is visible.
- IVP (page 48): an x-ray to outline the kidneys. A Wilm's tumour usually distorts the structure of the kidney. Tomograms (page 57) may be done to get better views of the tumour.
- A chest x-ray is routinely done to make sure that there has been no spread to the lungs.
- If required an arteriogram (page 54) may be done to outline the blood vessels in the kidney. This is a skilled procedure,

especially in young babies, and should only be done by those experienced in doing the test in babies.

- An ultrasound (page 59) of the abdomen may be useful in showing up a lump.
- Abdominal CT scans (page 59) are being more commonly used.
- Liver ultrasound (page 59) or isotope scan (page 62).
- Lung tomograms (page 57) or CT scan (page 59) to look for small amounts of tumour in the lungs.
- Bone scan (page 62) or bone x-ray.

This tumour may be confused with a neuroblastoma (page 256) of the adrenal gland, which lies just above the kidney, and a urine collection may be done to see if it contains catecholamines (page 257).

TREATMENT

The chances for cure of this common tumour are, fortunately, very good and because of this, and the complicated treatment necessary, children should be treated in a cancer centre.

The factors that affect the chance of cure are:

(1) Age, children under 2 years of age do better.
(2) Stage, the less the tumour has spread the better.
(3) The appearance of the tumour under a microscope.

Surgery (Chapter Twelve)

The key to cure is total removal of the tumour. This usually means taking out the affected kidney, an operation called a total nephrectomy. This operation should be done by an experienced paediatric surgeon as the operation needs careful planning and assessment of tumour spread. Many surgeons use metal clips to outline the site of the cancer in case radiotherapy is planned. Although in the past this operation was done as an emergency, it is much better to do it as a carefully planned procedure. If there are tumours affecting both kidneys it is often possible to remove the tumours and to leave enough unaffected kidney for the child to carry on a normal life. These children, of course, have to be looked after by specialists so that they very best operation can be planned.

Radiotherapy (Chapter Thirteen)

Radiation is often used together with surgery and may be given before or after an operation. If radiotherapy is given before an operation it may shrink the cancer down and make its removal easier, but there are also advantages for doing the operation first. The radiotherapy must be carefully planned to avoid over-treating normal tissues, especially the bones of the spine. Treatment is given 5 days each week for about 3 weeks. The first visit to the radiotherapy department is spent in planning the treatment which is individualized for each child. Most children have the radiotherapy after an operation and this is started within 1 to 5 weeks. They tolerate the radiotherapy well as high doses are not used. If the child has a tumour of both kidneys then great care in planning the radiation treatment is needed.

Chemotherapy (Chapter Fourteen)

On the whole these tumours respond well to drug treatment. Actinomycin D was the first drug to be used successfully and more recently adriamycin and vincristine have been used. Chemotherapy is often started soon after the operation to remove the tumour and is then given intermittently for a period of up to 15 months. An idea of the side-effects of the drugs to be used can be seen from looking up the drugs in Appendix A. The drugs used and the frequency and length of time for which they are given may vary from hospital to hospital and parents should discuss how this is to be done before treatment starts. Treatment is usually well tolerated apart from some sickness on the days when the drugs are given.

The total treatment plan must be designed for each individual case and it is not possible to give more than an outline of the typical methods of treatment. Although the treatment may seem complicated and to last for a long time most children are cured, so it is well worth it.

SUMMARY OF THE TREATMENT OF WILM'S TUMOUR

(1) The tumour is more common in some children with rare congenital abnormalities.

(2) Symptoms are few and many children are only found to have a tumour after their parents have noticed a lump in their abdomen, often at bath-time.

(3) A carefully planned operation to remove all or as much of the tumour as possible is important.

(4) This may be followed by radiotherapy to the site of the cancer, though if it is a large tumour the radiotherapy may be used to shrink the cancer before an operation.

(5) Chemotherapy is used to treat any cancer cells that may have spread and is often started soon after the operation and is continued for up to 18 months.

(6) This is a tumour that can be cured and should be treated in special cancer centres. The cure rate is about 80 per cent and even children with very advanced Wilm's tumour or with tumour of both kidneys can be cured.

(7) The whole family needs the support of a specialist team.

Notes

Soft tissue sarcomas

These are tumours of the soft parts of the body and the commonest type (rhabdomyosarcoma) arises in muscles. The treatment of this uncommon tumour has improved markedly in the last two decades so that about half of the children with this tumour are cured. This improvement has come from the use of combinations of surgery, radiotherapy, and chemotherapy. No cause is known and it does not run in families except in the rare cases of other conditions that can become a sarcoma (for instance von Recklinghausen's disease, Neurofibromatosis page 16).

SYMPTOMS

This tumour can start in any part of the body but is most common in the head and neck, the arms or legs, and in the genito-urinary tract (page 170). Because of this the symptoms that it may cause vary according to where the tumour is. The commonest symptom is swelling or a lump in a muscle. Though lumps and bruises are common and sarcomas are rare any child with a persistent lump in a muscle should be taken to a doctor. If a rhabdomyosarcoma is found the child should be treated in a specialist children's cancer centre.

DIAGNOSIS

A biopsy of the lump must be done to make sure of the diagnosis. Because these tumours tend to spread in lymphatics and the blood to other parts of the body a search must be made for metastases.
The following tests are used:

- Bone scan (page 62) to check the bones.
- CT scan of the chest and abdomen (page 59).
- Liver scan (page 63) or ultrasound (page 59) to look for spread to the liver.
- Bone marrow biopsy (page 66). This is done under a general anaesthetic in children.

Other tests will depend on where the tumour has started. If this is in the genito-urinary tract then tests may include:

- An IVP (page 48) to outline the kidneys, ureters, and bladder.
- Barium enema (page 46) to see if anything is pressing on to the large bowel.

If the tumour involves the head and neck extra information can be gained from these tests.

- X-ray of the skull to see if the bones of the skull are involved.
- Brain scan (page 65), CT scan (page 59) to check whether there is any spread inside the skull.
- Lumbar puncture (page 280) to check that there is no involvement of the fluid around the brain (CSF).

TREATMENT

Frequently surgery, radiotherapy, and chemotherapy are all used together to try to cure the child. Though the treatment is complex and difficult to tolerate, children are more resilient than adults and the 50 per cent chance of cure makes the side-effects worthwhile. Because these tumours can grow in so many different parts of the body it is not possible to give a definite pattern of treatment and the next sections only outline the general type of therapy that is used.

Surgery (Chapter Twelve)

The initial treatment consists of surgical removal of as much of the tumour as possible. The chances of doing this will depend on where the tumour is but every attempt is made to leave normal tissue and to get as good a cosmetic result as possible. Detailed discussion of the type of operation is beyond the scope of this book as it must be individualized for each child; parents must talk to the surgeon prior to any operation, as extensive surgery including amputation may be necessary.

Radiotherapy (Chapter Thirteen)

Radiotherapy is often given to the site of the tumour after as much as possible has been removed by an operation. High doses of radiotherapy may be required and treatment is divided into fractions given 4–5 days a week for 4 to 8 weeks. The side-effects of this treatment will, of course, depend on several factors including where the cancer is and before treatment starts parents should discuss the proposed programme and its side-effects. An idea of these may be gained from Chapter Thirteen. In some cases radiotherapy may be given before surgery in an attempt to make it possible to remove a tumour.

Chemotherapy (Chapter Fourteen)

Chemotherapy is often combined with local treatment either to deal with cancer that is known to have spread, or to treat suspected metastases even when none can be found (adjuvant treatment).

The drugs most commonly used are a combination of the following:

(1) Actinomycin D.
(2) Vincristine.
(3) Cyclophosphamide.
(4) Adriamycin.

A combination of these drugs is usually given at about 3-weekly intervals. The duration of treatment depends on whether the drugs are being given for metastatic disease or as an adjuvant for suspected disease. Parents will need to discuss the possible side-effects of treatment though most children are able to tolerate treatment better than adults. An idea of the toxicity of each of the drugs in a combination can be gained from looking up the individual drugs in Appendix A.

OUTLOOK

This depends on several factors.
• Site. Tumours developing in some parts of the body do comparatively better; these include tumours of the bladder, female genital tract, and around the eye.
• Stage. The chance of cure is clearly best in those with a small tumour that has not spread.
• Appearance under a microscope. The pattern the tumour forms varies and some (embryonal and botryoid) tumours do better than others.

268

- Age. Some studies have suggested that younger children have the best chance of cure.

SUMMARY OF THE TREATMENT OF
SOFT TISSUE SARCOMAS

(1) These tumours can affect many different parts of the body.
(2) Treatment and its side-effects will vary according to where the tumour is.
(3) At operation an attempt is made to remove all or as much as possible of the tumour and extensive surgery may be needed in some cases. Parents need to discuss the type of surgery and its consequences in detail.
(4) Radiotherapy may be used with surgery to treat the site of the tumour. High doses are often needed and these may cause side-effects and parents should discuss these. Radiotherapy may be given before or after an operation.
(5) Drug therapy (chemotherapy) is often given after local treatment. This may be given even if there is no evidence of disease spread, as there may be a high risk of microscopic deposits of tumour that we cannot see. Chemotherapy causes side-effects which need to be discussed before treatment.
(6) Despite the intensive type of treatments used for these tumours most children will tolerate the treatment reasonably well.
(7) The whole family will need the support of their own doctor and of a team of specialists during and after the treatment.
(8) This is a tumour that should be treated in a specialist cancer centre.

Notes

Chondrosarcoma

Unlike many of the bone tumours chrondrosarcomas often occur in middle life as well as in children. They tend to be slow growing and spread late in their course so that surgical removal is often curative. Some develop from pre-existing benign bone tumours called osteochondromas, enchonidromas, or chondromas.

They can grow anywhere and staging is mainly concerned with the extent of the primary tumour. The tests used include, plain x-rays, CT scans (page 59), and sometimes arteriograms (page 54).

TREATMENT

This is almost exclusively surgical. Most often the tumour and some surrounding bone are removed and this is all that is necessary. Occasionally if the tumour is large an amputation may be necessary. Surgery for this tumour should be done by someone experienced in the field as a common error is to do an inadequate removal of the cancer.

Notes

Ewing's sarcoma

This is a malignant tumour of bones that is most common between the ages of 5 to 16 years. Almost any bone can be involved and the tumour is more common in boys.

SYMPTOMS

As with other bone cancers the common symptoms are:

- Increasing and persistent pain over a bone.
- Swelling over bone.
- Decrease in movement if a limb bone is involved.

DIAGNOSIS

An x-ray will often show a swollen bone with an area of destruction. It is not always possible to be sure that this is a tumour and not infection or another disease. Because of this a biopsy (sample or a small piece of tissue) is always necessary.

If a cancer is suspected other investigations will include:

- A chest x-ray to make sure there has been no spread to the lungs. Lung tomograms (page 57) or a CT scan (page 59) may be done.
- A bone scan (page 62) or x-rays of other bones to see if the cancer has spread.
- A liver ultrasound (page 59) or isotope scan (page 63) may be used to examine the liver.
- A bone marrow biopsy (page 66) may be performed (under anaesthetic) to check for spread.

TREATMENT

As with most cancers in children a team of doctors is involved and children should be treated at a special cancer centre.

Surgery (Chapter Twelve)

Usually, the most important role of surgery in this tumour is to obtain a small piece (a biopsy) for microscopic examination. This is crucial to make the diagnosis and so that further treatment can be planned. The biopsy is usually taken from tumour in the soft tissue around the bone and is very rarely disfiguring. In most cases no further operation is needed though in certain parts of the body where it is difficult to cure the tumour with radiotherapy and drugs the place of an operation is being tested.

It is sometimes difficult to tell a Ewing's sarcoma from other tumours and pathologists may need to do special tests or to send the tissue biopsied to other pathologists. Because of this it may take some days to get an answer from the biopsy.

Radiotherapy (Chapter Thirteen)

This is usually the most important treatment. However, very high doses of radiation are needed and this treatment should only be done by experienced radiotherapists. Because of the high doses of radiotherapy it is important that a programme of active exercises is used during and after treatment to make sure that the function of the area treated is as good as possible. The first visit to the radiotherapy department is spent planning the individual treatment. The radiotherapy is then given for 4–5 days per week for 6–8 weeks. The immediate side-effects of treatment include soreness and reddening of the irradiated skin; this cannot be avoided because of the high dose being used and loose fitting clothes should be worn to avoid rubbing the skin. After radiotherapy, gradual thickening or scarring (fibrosis) of the skin occurs and unless physiotherapy exercises are conscienciously used then poor movement of joints can result.

Chemotherapy (Chapter Fourteen)

Radiotherapy is used to eradicate the local tumour, whereas drugs are used to treat cancer cells that have spread to other parts of the body. This is a very malignant tumour that frequently spreads and even if all tests are normal, treatment must be given for hidden disease (microscopic or micro-metastases). The drugs that are most often used are vincristine, cyclophosphamide, adriamycin, and actinomycin D. Treatment is given intermittently for some months and parents will need to discuss the type and duration of treatment before it starts.

The nature of combined radiotherapy–chemotherapy treatment will depend on several factors and treatment will have to be planned for each child. Radiotherapy may also be used locally to treat a tumour that has already spread to other parts of the body. The chances of cure have increased with modern management but unfortunately less than half the children treated will survive this tumour.

SUMMARY OF THE TREATMENT OF EWING'S SARCOMA

(1) This tumour of bones can arise anywhere.
(2) Surgery is usually only done to make the diagnosis.
(3) High doses of radiotherapy are used together with chemo- therapy.
(4) The cure rate has risen from 10 per cent to 40–50 per cent.
(5) Treatment should be given in a specialist centre.
(6) The whole family need the help and support of an experienced team.

Notes

Osteogenic sarcoma

This tumour of bone is most common between the ages of 10 to 25 years and is more prevalent in boys. Any bones in the body can be involved but the limb bones are most frequently affected.

SYMPTOMS

Pain and swelling of the involved part together with reduction in the use of the limb are the usual symptoms. A tender lump is often present and occasionally weight loss and malaise occur. Sometimes a weakened bone may break–a pathological fracture. Spread of the tumour is common and the lungs and other bones are most often involved.

DIAGNOSIS

An x-ray of the bone will usually show an area of destruction and thickening which may be typical for this tumour. If an x-ray shows this type of abnormality the child should be referred to a specialist cancer centre.

A sample of bone (biopsy) must be taken to make the diagnosis and before this is done more x-rays may be necessary. If the biopsy does shown an osteogenic sarcoma then further tests are needed to see if the tumour has spread. The tests include:

- Chest x-ray.
- Lung tomograms (page 57) or CT scan (page 59) to examine the lungs in greater detail.
- Bone scan (page 62).
- Liver scan (page 63).

TREATMENT

The treatment of this tumour has changed markedly in the past ten years. Before the 1970s surgery was the main treatment but despite amputations tumour developed in the lungs within a few months and the child died. This was because there were hidden cancer cells (micro- and microscopic metastases) in other parts of the body. Because of this, treatment now includes chemotherapy and/or radiotherapy.

Surgery

Because most tumours start in a limb bone operations in the past have usually meant removal of the affected part of the limb (an amputation). Though this sounds rather drastic it may be the only way of being sure of getting rid of the cancer and is often the best chance of survival. Recently, in certain cases, cancer centres have been testing whether extensive surgery (but not amputation) together with radiotherapy is as good as amputation. This is an experimental approach only available in a few special centres and although it usually means that the limb is saved a series of operations may be necessary and the limb is unlikely to function entirely normally. Parents must discuss the type of surgery recommended and its consequences in great detail. If an amputation is necessary it must be remembered that all these children will adapt well to an artificial limb and will, in most respects, be able to live a normal life. A programme of intensive rehabilitation should always be planned from the outset and can only be done by those experienced in this area of medicine.

Radiotherapy

Some centres use high doses of radiotherapy to shrink a tumour before an operation designed to preserve the limb. This type of treatment remains experimental and the effects of extensive surgery and radiation may mean that the limb does not work fully.

Chemotherapy

Most centres use combinations of chemotherapy drugs after surgery and/or radiotherapy. This is because of the very high risk of tumour spread (even if the usual tests are normal) in osteogenic sarcoma. The drugs most frequently used are methotrexate, adriamycin, vincristine, and cyclophosphamide and an idea of the side-effects of a regime can be gained from looking up the individual drugs in Appendix A. Treatment is usually given intermittently for 1 to 2 years and children usually feel sick and unwell for a few days with each treatment. Young children tolerate this well but teenagers find it is more difficult and if they have had an amputation have more problems adjusting.

If there is metastatic spread of the cancer chemotherapy is used, but surgical removal of tumour lumps (often from the lungs) is becoming more common and is curative in some cases.

OUTLOOK

The chances for cure have improved in the past 10 years from about 15 per cent to 40–50 per cent.

The factors affecting the prognosis are:

- Stage when diagnosed—the outlook is worse if there are already metastases.
- The microscopic appearance—a particular type of osteogenic sarcoma (paraosteal) is slower growing and 70–80 per cent of these patients are cured by an amputation alone.

SUMMARY OF THE TREATMENT OF OSTEOGENIC SARCOMA

(1) This is the commonest type of bone cancer and is most often seen between the ages of 10–25 years.
(2) Pain, swelling, and reduced movement of a limb are the most common symptoms.
(3) Investigations are done to see if the tumour has spread and a biopsy of the tumour must be done to confirm the diagnosis.
(4) Treatment should be in a special children's cancer centre.
(5) Amputation is the standard treatment but radiotherapy and/or chemotherapy may be used before an operation to preserve the limb; such an approach remains experimental.
(6) Intensive rehabilitation must be planned from the outset.
(7) Most centres use chemotherapy after surgery.
(8) Paraosteal sarcomas are slow growing and are usually curable with an amputation.
(9) Metastases are sometimes removed surgically (usually from the lungs) and such operations with chemotherapy can be curative.

(10) The chances of cure have risen from 15 per cent to 40–50 per cent.

(11) The whole family need the help and support of a full team of specialists.

Notes

Leukaemia

Leukaemia is cancer of the bone marrow cells, and in the past decade there have been great improvements in the methods of its treatment. There are several different types of leukaemia but only one of these, acute lymphocytic leukaemia (ALL), is common in children.

Aute lymphocytic leukaemia is, in fact, the commonest type of cancer in children, accounting for about one-third of all childhood cancers. It is most common between the age of 2 to 7 years and is uncommon after the age of 15.

As leukaemia is a cancer that grows in the bone marrow, where blood is made the leukaemic cells make it difficult for the body to form new blood. Because of this children become short of red cells (anaemic), white cells (becoming susceptible to infections), and the clotting cells called platelets (making them prone to bleeding).

SYMPTOMS

To begin with these are non-specific and include:

(1) Tiredness.
(2) Frequent infections that do not respond normally to antibiotics.
(3) Occasionally pain over the spleen (left side of abdomen).
Further symptoms that often develop are:

(4) Bruising, bleeding (particularly from the gums and nose), a rash consisting of tiny bleeding spots in the skin (petechae or purpura).
(5) Enlargement of lymph glands (page 36).
(6) Discovery of a lump in the abdomen (an enlarged spleen).
(7) Pain or discomfort over bones.

DIAGNOSIS

If leukaemia is suspected a routine blood count should be taken.

When leukaemia is found the count is usually abnormal. The changes in the count include:

(1) Anaemia (lack of red cells).
(2) A low white count due to a loss of normal cells, or a high white count because of leukaemic cells present in the blood.
(3) Lack of platelets (thrombocytopenia).

Although these abnormalities may strongly suggest leukaemia a bone marrow test (page 66) should always be done. In young children this is often done under a general anaesthetic and is best performed by those experienced in the treatment of leukaemia in children.

TREATMENT

Ideally all children with leukaemia (ALL) should be treated in a special children's cancer centre. This is a curable disease and every effort should be made to cure the child. The first stage of treatment is called 'remission induction'.

Remission induction

The first object of treatment is to get rid of all the leukaemic cells in the body. Drug treatment (chemotherapy) is used and two drugs, vincristine and prednisone, are the mainstay of treatment. They have far fewer side-effects than the types of treatment used for adult leukaemia. The major problem that children may notice is some 'pins and needles' in the fingers or feet; this is caused by vincristine and goes away after the treatment is stopped. During this early period of treatment children are at risk from infection or bleeding and must be watched closely. They may need to be in hospital during induction though most hospitals make every effort to get children home as soon as possible. Support with blood transfusions, antibiotics, and platelets transfusions may be needed to treat anaemia, infections, and bleeding respectively.

Over 90 per cent of children will be in complete remission (page 288) within one month. This does not mean they are cured, only that the leukaemia has been reduced to such an extent that it cannot be detected. All tests during a complete remission are normal and the child will feel much better. For the small proportion of children not in complete remission further treatment with other drugs is given.

Induction treatment for this type of leukaemia is, therefore, very successful and well tolerated though the child must be watched carefully for infection or bleeding. As soon as the child is in complete remission (CR) more treatment must be given to the brain and spinal cord.

Central nervous system prophylaxis

In the past up to half of children in complete remission developed leukaemia of the lining (meninges) of the brain and spinal cord. Because of this, treatment is given to prevent its occurrence (central nervous system prophylaxis) and is now an essential part of the treatment of childhood leukaemia. The treatment consists of radiotherapy to the head and a course of about five injections into the fluid in the spine (an intrathecal injection—page 56). The radiotherapy (Chapter Thirteen) is given about 4–5 times a week over about two weeks and causes *temporary* hair loss but is well tolerated. The intrathecal injections of a drug called methotrexate may be given under a general anaesthetic in young children, but should not be painful if performed skilfully. The combination of brain radiotherapy and intrathecal injections may cause temporary sleepiness but there are no obvious long term effects. After CNS prophylaxis it is normal to give maintenance drug treatment. Because there is a risk of leukaemia in the testis some hospitals give radiotherapy to the testicles to try to prevent this. This remains experimental but will always cause sterility. After the child has achieved a complete remission and has had CNS prophylactic treatment further chemotherapy, called maintenance treatment, is given.

Maintenance therapy

This usually consists of two or more drugs given by mouth in moderate doses. This is to remove any remaining microscopic collections of leukaemic cells. The doses are chosen so that they are well tolerated and the child is able to return to a normal life style.

However, regular blood counts are required to monitor the treatment and adjustments of the drug doses may be needed. Bone marrow examinations may be done every so often to check that all remains normal. The period of maintenance is usually at least 2 years and if the child has remained in complete remission all of this time the treatment is stopped altogether.

Viewed all at once the remission induction, CNS prophylaxis, and maintenance treatment seems a heavy programme for a child to cope with but if the treatment is completed the chances of cure is good.

Infection remains one of the problems throughout the treatment period. Any child undergoing treatment for leukaemia who develops signs of an infection should be seen by a doctor. These children do not have normal defence mechanisms and they respond badly to common infections, such as measles, and are more prone to unusual infections.

It is very important to try to protect these children from the common viral illnesses of childhood, such as chickenpox which may cause a fatal pneumonia in children being treated for leukaemia. Leukaemic children should live a normal life but must be isolated from friends and family who have an infection. Injections of immune serum can be given to children exposed to chickenpox infection but it is better to avoid contact with the infection. Prompt and expert treatment of any infection that does occur is important and most children will with appropriate treatment, recover.

RELAPSE

If the leukaemia returns it is said to have relapsed. It is usually possible to give further remission induction therapy and obtain a complete remission for a second, third, or even fourth time. However, the length of the remission gradually becomes shorter and few children with recurrent leukaemia live more than a few years. Recently, children relapsing with ALL are being considered for a bone marrow transplantation and this may offer a small chance of cure.

SUPPORT

In addition to the expertise in treating leukaemia a children's cancer centre can provide the emotional and practical support that is most important for the family of the child with leukaemia. The period of treatment is long and fraught with difficulty and even with complete remission the future is uncertain. This is tough for

282

parents and hard to come to terms with, but with experienced medical staff problems can be recognized and discussed and appropriate support given.

THE CHANCES OF CURE

About half of all patients with childhood acute lymphocytic leukaemia can be cured with current treatment. The risk of relapse is highest in the two years after stopping treatment and the risk then gets progressively less. This greatly improved chance of cure has only come from the careful use of all the treatments described.

SUMMARY OF THE TREATMENT OF CHILDHOOD ACUTE LYMPHOCYTIC LEUKAEMIA

(1) The commonest symptoms are of tiredness, infections, bleeding, and enlarged lymph nodes.
(2) The first stage of treatment is remission induction. Vincristine and prednisone are usually used and the treatment is well tolerated.
(3) The child may need hospitalization for part of this period.
(4) Over 90 per cent of children have a complete remission.
(5) The next step is CNS prophylaxis. Radiotherapy is given to the brain together with a course of intrathecal injections.
(6) Following this, two or more years maintenance drug therapy is given. Infections are a risk during maintenance.
(7) If there has been no relapse, treatment is then stopped. The risk of relapse is highest in the first two years.
(8) The chance of cure is about 50 per cent.

283

Notes

Lymphomas

The treatment and outlook of children with lymphomas is sometimes different from that of adults and they are considered separately in this section.

HODGKIN'S DISEASE

The risk of Hodgkin's disease is very low in babies but gradually rises in childhood to reach a peak in the twenties. The spread of this disease and its staging is the same as in adults (page 202). The investigations used to find out the extent of the disease include:

- Chest x-ray and possibly lung tomograms (page 57).
- Lymphangiogram (page 51).
- Full blood count and biochemical tests on the blood.
- Bone marrow examination (page 66).
- Liver and bone scans (pages 63 and 62).

In adults an exploratory operation including removal of the spleen (staging laparotomy—page 204) is usually carried out in patients being considered for radiotherapy rather than chemotherapy. However, more children are now being routinely treated with a combination of radiotherapy and chemotherapy and the operation is becoming less important. Many hospitals do not, therefore, use a staging laparotomy and will go straight ahead with combined therapy. The chances of cure are good with this cancer but are affected by the stage, as in adults.

TREATMENT

It is important to avoid giving a large dose of radiotherapy to growing bones and for this reason low doses are used together with chemotherapy even in patients with apparently localized disease. This has the added advantage that a staging laparotomy is less important and is useful because there is a risk of infection after removal of the spleen. A treatment plan will be designed for each child and parents will need to discuss the details of the treatment before it starts. The chapters on radiotherapy, chemotherapy, and adult Hodgkin's disease will suggest some questions and the following list may be helpful.

(1) Is a staging laparotomy being considered?
(2) Is radiotherapy or chemotherapy or a combination of both to be used.
(3) What are the immediate side-effects of treatment?
(4) How long will the treatment take?
(5) Are there any long-term effects of treatment?
(6) Does the treatment affect fertility?
(7) What are the chances of cure?

As with all childhood cancers it is desirable that the child should be treated in a special centre.

NON-HODGKIN'S LYMPHOMA

As in adults there are numerous different types of non-Hodgkin's lymphoma. However, most fall into the group of more rapidly growing and potentially curable lymphomas.

Symptoms

Children can develop many different symptoms but several groups of symptoms are typical.

- Tumour in the chest, around the heart may cause shortness of breath, glands in the neck, and fluid in the chest (a pleural effusion—page 69). There may be involvement of the bone marrow.
- Disease in the digestive tract. The small bowel and stomach are most frequently involved. Children may develop stoppages of the bowel (bowel obstruction) and the diagnosis is often only made at an operation to find the cause of obstruction.
- Disease of lymph nodes in the abdomen. Children may develop greatly enlarged abdominal lymph nodes which can be felt as lumps. There may be no obvious disease outside the abdomen and an exploratory operation (a laparotomy) may be needed to make the diagnosis.
- Enlarged lymph nodes. Other children may develop enlarged nodes in the neck, groins, or under the arms. Often the nodes are confined to one of these areas.

- Tonsil or adenoid involvement. Lymphoma of these glands is often associated with enlarged lymph nodes in the neck. Occasionally it is associated with involvement of the stomach or bowel.

Investigation and treatment

Because of the differing patterns of spread and of types of lymphoma it is too complicated to give more than an outline of treatment.

Investigations will vary from child to child but may include:

- Chest x-ray.
- Lymphangiogram (page 51).
- Full blood count and biochemical tests on the blood.
- Bone marrow examination (page 66).
- Liver and bone scans (pages 63 and 62).
- An explanatory operation may be needed to make the diagnosis in cases of bowel obstruction or in disease confined to the abdomen.

Treatment varies from hospital to hospital but will be based on common principles. Because most of these lymphomas are of a fast growing type the treatment is intensive with several drugs used (combination chemotherapy) to try to eradicate all traces of the cancer. This may be combined with radiation therapy and is often followed by a period of less intensive maintenance chemo-therapy (see section on childhood leukaemia—page 280) for up to two years. There is also an increased risk of lymphoma of the lining of the brain with certain types of childhood lymphoma and CNS prophylactic x-ray therapy and drugs (page 280) may be needed, as in leukaemic children. The treatment is often compli-cated and the side-effects and duration of treatment may seem formidable but the good chance of cure makes it worthwhile. As in leukaemia families need total support during treatment and care in a special children's cancer centre is preferable.

SUMMARY OF THE TREATMENT OF CHILDHOOD LYMPHOMA

(1) There are several types of lymphoma in children. Most are fast growing.

(2) There are several patterns of lymphoma including spread in the chest, stomach or bowel, lymph nodes in the abdomen, lymph nodes in the rest of the body, and lymphoma of the tonsils.

(3) Investigations are done to 'stage' the disease. An exploratory abdominal operation may be needed to make the diagnosis in some children.

(4) Treatment mainly uses chemotherapy though radiotherapy may also be used in certain children.

(5) Treatment, in some lymphomas, may be given to prevent spread to the brain.

(6) If a complete remission is achieved, maintenance treatment is often given for about two years.

(7) In some children the chance of cure is good if treatment is carefully planned and administered.

Notes

CHAPTER SEVENTEEN

What are response, relapse, and remission?

Medical language is hard to follow, this chapter aims to explain some of the terms used when talking about the way a cancer responds to treatment and of how well patients do.

RESPONSE OR REMISSION

These words are used to describe a reduction in the size of tumour. The proportion (per cent) of patients who achieve a response is called the response rate. Responses may be of two main types.

- Partial response or remission (PR) is usually defined as a reduction in the size of a 'measurable' tumour that is greater than half (50 per cent) and lasts for at least one month. There is, however, still detectable tumour. Shrinkage of tumour that is less than half is usually disregarded by doctors as not being of sufficient benefit. A partial response rate is the proportion of patients whose tumour shrinks to less than half of its previous size.
- Complete response or remission (CR). This is complete disappearance of a tumour so that it is not detectable on examination or after repeating all tests that were previously abnormal. Occasionally, as in ovarian cancer (page 148) there may be a second operation to ensure that there is no remaining tumour. A complete remission does **not** mean cure. It only indicates that there is no tumour that can be seen using our present day tests. If there are even a few surviving cancer cells then they may grow back so that the tumour eventually reappears. A complete response rate is the proportion of patients achieving a complete remission.
- Overall response rate is a term used to combine the partial and complete responders. It is the proportion of patients who have a complete response or shrinkage of their tumour by at least a half.

RELAPSE

If a patient who has gained a complete remission then has the tumour grow back they are said to have relapsed. Relapse does not imply that further treatment is not helpful and in some cancers a second complete remission and cure is still possible.

PROGRESSION

Progression is a term implying that a tumour has continued to grow despite treatment. It may also be used to describe a tumour which starts to grow again after a partial response.

SURVIVAL

When treatments are being tested in trials the length of time that patients survive is often quoted. The figure that is usually given is the length of time that has elapsed when half the patients have died. This is shown graphically in Figure 43 and is called the *median survival* time. In this example when only half (50 per cent) of the patients are surviving the length of time of survival is 200 days. This does not mean that all patients will survive 200 days. Indeed half (50 per cent) of the patients have died within 200 days and half survive longer than this (in Figure 43 about 20 per cent are alive at 500 days and some may be cured).

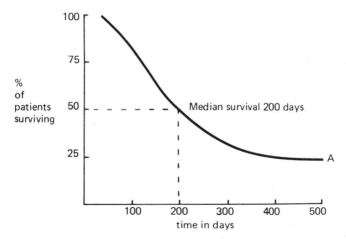

Figure 43 Median survival: if there are a hundred patients with a cancer it is the length of time the person who is the 50th to die survives

290

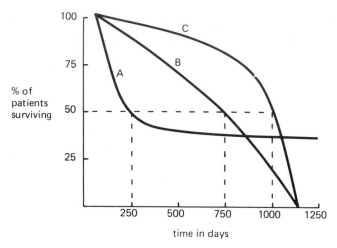

Figure 44 Median survival: this does not say anything about the curability of a cancer. In this graph patients in group A have a short median survival (250 days) whilst patients in groups B and C do better (median survival 750 and 1000 days). However, all the patients in groups B and C are dead by 1200 days whilst about 40 per cent of group A are alive and possibly cured

Survival is nearly always discussed in these terms but this can be very misleading and Figure 44 shows how a false impression can be given by only talking about a median survival. Patients receiving treatment A only have a median survival of 250 days, but more importantly about 40 per cent are alive at 1250 days and are probably cured. Patients in group B have a much better median survival (750 days) but none are cured and all are dead by 1100 days. In group C few die early and the median survival is excellent (1000 days); however, after two years many patients die and all are dead by 1100 days. Although the median survival is worst in group A is it amongst these patients that the best chance for cure lies.

When the results of treatment are discussed it is important to look at the shape of a surival curve and not just a median survival. When survival is talked about it is important to remember that the chances of survival depend on many factors including the appearance of the tumour under a microscope, the extent of spread (stage, page 40), and the general health of the patient. Information on survival should be related to the important factors that are known to influence the patient's outlook. However, doctors can never give an accurate estimate of how long a patient will live as everybody is different. Most doctors are reluctant to say how a patient will do and any figure given must be taken as approximate.

RELAPSE-FREE SURVIVAL (Progression free interval)

This is a term that only applies to patients who achieve a complete remission. It is the time from the start of treatment till the disease relapses.

CURE

It may seem odd that it is difficult to define cure. The proper definition is that the survival of a group of patients is the same as a similar group of people who do not have the cancer that is being studied. In other words the patients with cancer die of other diseases at the same rate as a normal population. This definition can never be usefully applied as it takes very many years to gather such information.

Instead, cure is usually talked about in terms of lack of tumour *relapse* over a defined period of time. Although there are often no clear guide-lines this period of time varies from tumour to tumour. Thus, in the case of testicular teratomas a two-year period without relapse is regarded by many cancer specialists as tantamount to cure. For Hodgkin's diseas a five-year period is required whilst in breast cancer relapses can occur after ten years and a fifteen or twenty-year period may be necessary before cure can be talked about. Despite this it is true of all cancers that the risk of relapse is greatest in the first year after stopping treatment and with each succeeding year the risk diminishes.

CHAPTER EIGHTEEN

Treatment for the symptoms of cancer
with Susan Williams

Cancer may cause all sorts of different symptoms depending on which part of the body it affects. As well as specific treatment to reduce or get rid of the tumour other treatments can be used to treat the symptoms. Both approaches should be used together, though in very advanced cases it may be best to rely on treatment of the symptoms only.

Because anticancer treatment often causes side-effects (Chapters Twelve to Fourteen) it is sometimes necessary to use other drugs to try to reduce these effects. Treatment of symptoms, therefore, is very important.

PAIN CONTROL

Most people associate cancer with a painful progressive illness that ends in death. In fact about one-half of patients with _advanced_ cancers have no significant pain. For those patients who do have pain expert care is important.

One of the most important reasons for failure to control pain is a lack of appreciation by doctors that it is not a simple physical sensation. As well as the physical perception of pain there is an emotional reaction to it. Perception of pain and pain thresholds are, therefore, closely linked to mood and morale and a good relationship between patient and doctor is very helpful. Pain is extremely difficult to evaluate. It varies from person to person, some people can tolerate a lot more than others without requesting some kind of relief. It is hard to describe; 'like toothache', a 'stabbing feeling', a 'sharp pain', a 'dull ache'. It is even difficult to sometimes point to exactly where the pain is: a good guide for doctors evaluating cancer pain is that 'the pain is what the patients says it is'. Pain-killers are especially helpful at this time and the right dose, to ensure complete relief without causing drowsiness, needs expert care. A patient and doctor should work together to achieve this maxim.

Description of pain

It is very difficult to describe the quality of a pain though descriptions like 'a gnawing toothache' or 'a stabbing pain' can be helpful. Because it may be difficult for a patient to say exactly where a pain is many doctors ask patients to draw in the area of pain on a picture of the body.

Pain often varies in intensity during the day though this is sometimes due to the use of drugs which ease pain for an hour or so and then allow the pain to return before the next dose. Pain at night may also be worse than during the day as the person is more likely to feel alone at this time and may not take pain-killers at night. If a pain is worse on movement or weight bearing this is useful information for a doctor.

A pain may be chronic or acute. Chronic pain can become all consuming and it has:

- No foreseeable end.
- It tends to get worse not better.
- It serves no purpose.
- It takes up all the patient's attention and can make life not worth living.

Such pain requires expert treatment and in most cases it is possible to control it and make life worthwhile again.

Use of pain-killing drugs (analgesics)

The key to successfully controlling pain is to make sure that it is kept at bay all the time. For this reason it is wrong to delay taking a pain medicine until the pain has come back and is bad again. Continuous pain logically requires continuous treatment, so regular doses of drugs which prevent the pain returning should be used. Some doctors still prescribe pain killers 'to be taken as required'—this is not helpful, except in intermittent pain, as the drug *must* be taken before the pain returns. If after taking a pain killer a patient is pain free for 4 to 5 hours then she will need to take her next tablet after about 3½ hours. Most pain-killers work for approximately 4 hours if given in the correct dose. Hence it is logical to take it about every 4 hours even if the pain has not returned.

Pain at night can be a problem and sometimes it is better to wake in the middle of the night (set an alarm) for the next dose rather than be awoken by pain a little later and not get back to sleep. Once pain has returned it takes longer to get under control and often increasing doses of pain-killers are needed. Although many patients and even doctors worry about taking medicines, regular and adequate doses of pain-killers are essential and safe if used correctly. Doctors are more and more aware of this and so the standard of pain control has improved even in the past ten years.

Choice of pain-killer

This will depend on the severity of the pain and treatment starts with the simplest drug likely to be useful.

(1) Mild pain

This can be controlled by aspirin or paracetamol (panadol). Regular use of 1 or 2 tablets every 4–6 hours is recommended and many patients can tolerate up to 4 tablets of aspirin every 4 hours. However, patients receiving chemotherapy or those with a low blood count should try to avoid aspirin as it damages the platelets (page 101).

(2) Moderate pain

When aspirin and paracetamol fail then weak narcotic drugs are used. The most useful is often a combination of drugs including a codeine derivative. The commonly used drugs (brand names) include:

   (1) Distalgesic (containing paracetamol and dextropropoxyphene).
   (2) Napsalgesic (containing aspirin and dextropropoxyphene).
   (3) Codis (containing aspirin and codeine phosphate).
   (4) Paracodal (containing paracetamol and codeine).
   (5) DF118 (containing dihydrocodeine tartrate).

(6) Paramol–118 (containing paracetamol and dihydrocodeine tartrate).

The usual dose is 1 or 2 tablets taken regularly every 4–6 hours.

(3) Severe pain

This requires much stronger drugs and narcotics are usually given. These are a group of opium-like substances that are powerful pain-killers. When used for severe pain, they do not result in drug addiction or dependence. Unfortunately, many patients, nurses, and doctors do not realize this. It is always worth using these drugs when pain is severe and not uncommonly the dose can be reduced once the pain is controlled. There are various ways of giving narcotic drugs and several preparations. It is nearly always best to give the drug by mouth though injections may rarely be better for a few patients. The preparations that are available include:

(1) Nepenthe (with or without aspirin): a mixture of opium alkaloids with a measured amount of morphine.

(2) Morphine syrup ⎫ these may be mixed with alcohol or
(3) Diamorphine syrup ⎬ a fruit drink and only differ in
  ⎭ potency.

(4) MST–1: a slow release morphine in a special tablet.
(5) Buprenorphine: a new pain-killer for moderate pain.

Other drugs (brand names) similar in strength can be used.

(6) Palfium: potent but short-acting.
(7) Narphen: a potent alternative to diamorphine less likely to cause nausea—not available as a liquid.
(8) Dromoran: a potent short-acting alternative.

These strong drugs cannot be bought at a chemist's shop and can only be prescribed by a doctor.

Overwhelming pain requires urgent medical treatment and the most effective way of dealing with the pain is to give injections of a narcotic pain-killer (usually diamorphine) together with a sedative such as valium. This can be repeated, with increasing doses, every 1 to 2 hours until the pain is controlled. The patient, who will be exhausted anyway, may then sleep for long periods and when the pain has been controlled for several days the doses may be reduced and the drugs given less frequently by mouth.

This is not an exhaustive list of pain drugs and many patients may be given different drugs and it should be remembered that the drug names may vary by country. It is also worth knowing that most drugs have a proper name and a drug company (proprietary) name.

Whichever drugs are used it is the regular use of the pain-killer *before* pain returns that is paramount.

Other drugs that may be used together with pain-killers

Various drugs useful for anxiety or depression may be added to pain-killers. This helps by reducing the psychological part of the pain as well as by increasing the power of the pain-killer. The drugs (proprietary names) that may be used include:

(1) Largactil (chlorpromazine)
(2) Valium and other antianxiety drugs.
(3) Many different antidepressants.
(4) Sleeping tablets at night.

Steroids can also be beneficial and prednisolone tablets may be given with pain-killers for certain specific pains. In addition they often have a non-specific effect of making patients feel better, increase appetite, and lift mood. Drugs usually used for rheumatic conditions (anti-inflammatory drugs) may also be given with pain-killers especially if the pain is in a bone or caused by pressure on a nerve.

Other ways of controlling pain

(1) Pain sensations are carried by nerves and it is often possible to stop (block) the nerve from carrying the pain impulses to the brain. This can be done by injecting local anaesthetic near to the nerve (as a dentist does) or by using an injection which damages the nerve permanently. These techniques are specialized and patients need to discuss their use, but they should be available in most general hospitals. They are less useful for cancer pain than for chronic pain of other causes.

(2) Hypnosis is only an adjunct to other methods of treating pain. It produces an altered state of consciousness—even in difficult subjects and helps them to control their own pain. Whilst this may be successful in some patients it is not commonly used but often its great value is that a doctor will spend half an hour with them.

(3) Acupuncture. Though this would seem, by anecdote, to be a useful treatment it remains to be tested in cancer patients. Its disadvantage is that the effect does not last long.

(4) Peripheral nerve stimulation. Electrical stimulation of the skin near painful areas may reduce pain. This is most effective if the result lasts after the stimulation has stopped.

(5) Nitrous oxide gas mixtures. Very severe short lasting pains are difficult to deal with and some hospitals get patients to breathe an anaesthetic gas mixture, nitrous oxide, when they get a spasm of pain. The effect comes on quickly and passes off quickly and it may occasionally be useful for short but severe pains, e.g. if turning in bed hurts a patient or changing a dressing causes discomfort.

The control of pain is complex and patients with severe pain often need the help of a doctor skilled in this field. The important points to remember are:

- Pain is not only physical—every effort should be made to deal with anxiety and depression and patients should be given an opportunity to discuss their condition.
- If drugs are used they must be taken regularly so that the pain does not return between doses.
- If pain is severe narcotic drugs are needed, these will not cause addiction.
- Other methods of pain control are available.
- Substantial pain control can almost always be achieved.

CONSTIPATION

Constipation can be more troublesome than pain for patients with cancer. It is probably due to change in diet, loss of appetite, chemotherapy, depression, unaccustomed inactivity perhaps, and most importantly, the use of pain-killing drugs. It is important to consider ways of dealing with this and doctors will probably recommend a laxative, which with sensible use will help.

Laxatives may be of several types.

(1) Purgatives such as senna that work by stimulating the bowel.
(2) Stool softeners such as liquid paraffin and drugs that increase the bulk.
(3) Other drugs, such as Dorbanex Medro, are a combination of these drugs and work both ways. If purgatives are given alone they may cause colicky pain and it is usually best to give a stool softener as well. If after 3 days, laxatives have failed to work, then further treatment is required and suppositories are commonly used, though it may become necessary to give an enema. People, even in good health, can become unnecessarily preoccupied with their bowel habits and worry about quite insignificant constipation.

DIARRHOEA

This may be a symptom of the cancer or a side-effect of its treatment. The best antidiarrhoreal drugs are codeine phosphate tablets (1 or 2, three times a day) and lomotil (1 or 2, four times a day). They are both effective and can be used together in severe cases and act by prolonging bowel transit and increasing fluid absorption.

NAUSEA AND VOMITING

This may be caused by the cancer but is also very common after chemotherapy (Chapter Fourteen) and radiotherapy (Chapter Thirteen) If the nausea and vomiting are severe it may be necessary to start treatment with injections of antisickness drugs (antiemetics) as any pills will be vomited back.

The drugs used (injection or tablets) include the following (trade name in brackets):

Chlorpramazine (Largactil
Prochlorperazine (Stemetil) } acting mainly on the brain.
Promazine (Sparine)
Cyclizine (Marzine)
Metoclopramide (Maxolon) — acting mainly on the bowel

They may be used alone or in combination since they act in different parts of the body or brain and usually control nausea caused by the cancer. It is more difficult to prevent the vomiting caused by anticancer chemotherapy and new antisickness drugs are being tested. Most antisickness drugs can be used every 4–6 hours and the next tablet should be taken before the sickness returns. Because they may cause drowsiness patients should avoid driving whilst on these drugs.

LOSS OF APPETITE

Loss of appetite and weight is very common in all sorts of cancer and may be due to several factors:

(1) Poor appetite causing a reduction in the patient's intake of calories and protein.
(2) The tumour altering the body's metabolism and 'burning' up excessive amounts of energy.
(3) Symptoms of the cancer (or its treatment), such as nausea and vomiting, diarrhoea, and failure to absorb food that is eaten, can all contribute to weight loss.

Prolonged loss of appetite (anorexia) leads to wasting which is known as cachexia. The symptoms of this condition, which is common in advanced cancer, are:

- Increasing emaciation.
- Generalized and progressive weakness.
- Loss of appetite — the thought or smell of food usually revolts the patient.
- Changes in the body's hormones.

The condition is difficult to treat because a vicious circle develops; the more the patient loses weight the less they want to eat. Relatives are concerned and often press patients to eat a normal meal in order to make them 'stronger' but this is usually rejected. It is better that they eat small meals of anything they may fancy. In addition many patients have poor or altered taste so that even when they feel hungry they may be dissuaded by the smell of food. Food that looks good but which does not have a strong smell may be acceptable to these patients. 'Tasty' foods are usually preferred to bland foods.

The use of alcohol or 'tonics' before meals may help improve appetite but the only generally successful treatment is the use of steroids. Prednisone tablets will increase appetite and often improve mood and make patients generally feel better. Food supplements containing protein and with a high calorie content may also be useful. They can be obtained in various flavours although many patients find them tasteless. The names of commercial preparations vary from country to country and include:

UK	USA
Build-up★	Sustacal
Caloreen	Meritene
Casilan	Lanolac
Clinifeed★	
Hycal	

★ Patients usually find these most palatable.

In patients who are likely to respond to anticancer treatment infusions of special high calorie and protein mixtures may occasionally be given into a vein. This is known as intravenous hyperalimentation and it is used to build up a patient who is already weak or ill. It must be done in hospital and a fine plastic catheter (tube) is usually put into a vein in the neck. It is the surest way of feeding up a patient but is only justified if the patient's cancer is being treated, as it is complicated.

DRY MOUTH

This is a common symptom that is often due to a combination of factors. The commonest of these are:

- Certain drugs, especially pain-killers, antidepressants, sedatives, and antisickness drugs.
- Radiotherapy to the neck or jaws.
- Decreased body fluids (dehydration).
- Poor appetite.
- Mouth breathing.

Sometimes the treatment that is causing the dry mouth can be stopped but usually it is only possible to try to increase the patient's saliva. Patients can do this by sucking acid sweets (such as lemon drops) or chewing gum. If the problem is severe, artificial saliva can be prescribed by a doctor and dehydrated patients can be helped by replacing their lost fluids.

SORE MOUTH

This may also be due to a variety of causes:

- Fungus infections (monilia, or thrush).
- Drug reactions (Appendix A and Chapter Fourteen).
- Aphthous ulcers.
- Vitamin deficiencies.
- Bacterial infections.
- Cold sores (herpes simplex).

Patients whose normal immunity is reduced are prone to get a fungal infection called monilia (thrush). Steroids, antibiotics, and anticancer drugs all increase the risk of this infection and as all three types of drugs are used in cancer patients it is not surprising that monilia mouth infections are common.

Careful cleansing of the mouth is, therefore, very important in order to avoid or reduce the problem. Teeth should be cleaned 3–4 times a day with a soft toothbrush and at times of high risk dentures should be removed except for meals. Non-alcohol containing mouth-washes should be used 3–4 times a day (see page 89). Corsodyl (containing the antiseptic chlorhexadine), oraldene and betadine mouth-washes are commercial preparations that are available. Diflam oral rinse is an anaesthetic mouth-wash which is useful for reducing the discomfort.

If a fungal infection does develop then antifungal lozenges and mouth-washes must be used. The treatments (brand name in brackets) used include:

(1) Amphoteracin (Fungilin) lozenges, which should be dissolved slowly in the mouth or suspension which is used as a mouth-wash then swallowed. Both should be used at least 4 times a day.
(2) Miconazole (Daktarin) gel which is used to rinse the mouth at least 4 times a day.
(3) Nystatin (Nystatin) suspension used to rinse the mouth at least 4 times a day.
(4) Ketoconazole a new drug which is absorbed into the body.

Aphthous ulcers are small painful ulcers that develop on the gums and inside the lips. They can occur in anyone at any time but are more common at times of stress or illness. Hydrocortisone lozenges (Corlan) can be useful if they are held in the mouth against the ulcer. Carbenoxolone, known as Bioral gel, can also be applied to an ulcer, as can Bonjela which can deaden pain.

Only rarely do vitamins improve a sore mouth but if there is a specific vitamin deficiency they will be helpful. Anticancer drugs may damage the lining (mucosa) of the mouth and temporary soreness and ulceration are common. Good hygiene is important and if no bacterial or fungal infection develops this will recover after 4–7 days. If a sore mouth is caused by the drug methotrexate (see Appendix A) then folinic acid mouth-washes help healing.

DIFFICULTY IN SWALLOWING

If there is narrowing of the oesophagus (gullet) or if a tumour presses on the oesophagus this causes difficulty in swallowing (called dysphagia). Though some cancers can respond quickly to chemotherapy or radiotherapy the majority that commonly cause difficulty in swallowing do not. An operation to insert a special tube through the tumour is often very helpful (page 127) and allows the patient to eat normally once again.

Not all patients with difficulty in swallowing have tumour in or pressing on the gullet and it is important to find out why this has happened. Sometimes fungal infections of the mouth (candida) spread down the oesophagus and cause painful difficulty in swallowing.

OBSTRUCTION OF THE BOWEL (intestinal obstruction)

Obstruction or blockage of the bowel is most often caused by cancer of the large bowel but is also common in ovarian cancer. It usually starts slowly with occasional episodes of colicky pain in the abdomen. A colicky pain comes and goes, like the pain we may get if we eat too many green apples. The pain is often accompanied by loud bowel sounds, swelling of the abdomen and sometimes diarrhoea. The symptoms of complete bowel obstruction are:

- Colicky abdominal pain.
- Nausea.

- Then vomiting.
- Constipation which becomes so complete that even wind is not passed.
- Waves of muscular contractions in the bowel that may occasionally be visible through the wall of the abdomen.

Anyone with these symptoms should be seen by a doctor immediately and if there is complete bowel obstruction they will usually need to be treated in hospital. Initially the bowel is rested by stopping the patient eating any food and fluids, they are then given fluids by an intravenous infusion (drip) into the vein. If nausea or vomiting is severe then a tube (nasogastric tube) is passed through the nose into the patient's stomach and the excess fluids are sucked off. This is mildly uncomfortable but rapidly relieves any nausea. In many cases the obstruction will settle with this simple treatment. If it does not then surgery will be considered to relieve the problem. Such operations are usually confined to patients with a cancer of the large bowel but usually mean that a colostomy (pages 131 and 326) is necessary. If the cancer cannot be operated on then radiotherapy (page 84) or chemotherapy (page 93) can occasionally be helpful. Even if these treatments are not useful, intravenous fluids (drip), and suction of the stomach contents will often 'settle' the blockage down and when used together with pain-killers and antisickness drugs can remove the unpleasant symptoms.

If the cancer is very advanced, operations, nasogastric tubes, and infusions may not be necessary as drugs can provide relief without the need for any unpleasant or distressing treatment. The treatment of intestinal obstruction depends entirely on the extent of the tumour.

- If the patient is not known to have cancer they will require an operation to make the diagnosis and this may be curative if there is only a localized bowel cancer.
- Patients with recurrent or progressive disease. If the patient has bowel cancer affecting one part of the bowel only, an operation can provide good relief but is rarely curative. In the case of recurrent ovarian cancer operations are rarely helpful and other treatments should be considered.
- For some patients there will be no treatment that can control the tumour but it is important to remember that treatment can be used to help the symptoms.

Abdominal pains, nausea, and bowel upsets are common in patients with cancer and are usually *not* due to an obstruction. However, patients with the symptoms mentioned above should seek medical advice early.

COLLECTION OF FLUID IN THE ABDOMEN (ascites)

Sometimes a tumour in the abdomen causes fluid to accumulate and this can lead to uncomfortable swelling and difficulty in breathing like that in pregnancy. The discomfort can be eased quickly by aspirating (drawing off) the fluid. A narrow plastic tube (catheter) is inserted through the skin of the abdomen (after local anaesthetic) and the fluid is sucked up into a syringe or a suction bottle. This may take several hours but is relatively painless and dramatically relieves the symptoms.

Sometimes a drug, usually bleomycin (Appendix A), is injected through the tube to try to prevent the fluid returning. If possible, specific anticancer treatment, radiotherapy, or chemotherapy should also be used to stop reaccumulation of the ascites. The procedure is mildly uncomfortable and is usually done in hospital.

INCREASED CALCIUM IN THE BLOOD (hypercalcamia)

Calcium is a salt normally held in bones and teeth which can be released into the blood in large quantities in some cancers. When there are increased amounts of calcium in the blood it has the following effects:

- It may cause constipation.
- Nausea and vomiting.
- Loss of appetite.
- Drowsiness and confusion.
- Weakness.

Treatment is to give large quantities of fluid, usually as an intravenous infusion (drip). If this does not reduce the high level of calcium, steroids are given and is usually successful. Other drugs can be used if these steps do not reduce the calcium level.

It is also important to try to plan therapy to shrink the cancer itself. The only sure way to get rid of the symptoms of hypercalcaemia is to get rid of the cause of the raised calcium — the cancer.

Unless a patient is really very ill, admission to hospital for a short period is advisable if hypercalcaemia develops. The use of infusions and steroids will get rid of the symptoms and anticancer treatment can be planned.

SHORTNESS OF BREATH

Shortness of breath, often with a cough, is not uncommon in advanced cancer. There are many possible causes, many unrelated to the cancer, but the commonest are:

- Tumour in the lung.
- Development of a collection of fluid in the chest (a pleural effusion).
- Scarring of the lungs after radiation or chemotherapy.
- Severe anaemia.
- Infection in the lung.

If there is tumour in the lung then treatment will need to be specific anticancer therapy, usually chemotherapy or radio-therapy. When a pleural effusion develops the shortness of breath it causes can be improved by draining off the fluid (pleural aspiration).

This may be done in two ways:

(1) If the fluid has not previously been troublesome then a thin needle is passed through the chest wall (between the ribs) into the fluid (page 69). The fluid is removed using a syringe or suction bottle and the needle is then taken out. The procedure is performed after the injection of a local anaesthetic and takes about half an hour.

(2) If the fluid keeps returning then a small operation is performed to put a plastic tube (catheter) into the chest. This is done under local anaesthetic and only takes a few minutes. The plastic catheter is then connected to a bottle with water in it — this stops air getting back into the chest and the fluid in the chest is slowly sucked out until none is left. A drug is then injected through the tube into the chest to stop the fluid coming back. This type of treatment is successful in over half of the cases and is well worth trying.

Patients will be in hospital for about 2–3 days. The tube may be mildly uncomfortable and can interfere with sleep whilst it is in the chest, but is it removed once the fluid has been taken away and the injection given.

- Inflammation of the lungs may occasionally occur several months after radiation has been given to the chest but is much less common today than it was. It is often accompanied by a cough and feeling of being generally unwell. The way to deal with it is to give steroids which relieves the inflammation and symptoms. The dose of steroids (usually prednisone tablets) must be reduced very gradually as the problem often returns if they are stopped suddenly. Shortness of breath developing some years after radiotherapy and caused by radiation scarring (fibrosis) is more difficult to treat and cannot be reversed.
- Severe anaemia is easily treated with a blood transfusion and patients often feel much better afterwards. Most patients are not short of iron and iron tablets are usually not helpful. Infections are common (page 101) and require treatment with antibiotics but viruses or any other unusual infections can be difficult to treat.

COUGH

If a cough is caused by a specific problem that can be treated (for instance, bronchitis treated with antibiotic) this is the most important aspect of treatment. If a curative treatment is not available 'cough mixtures' (antitussives) are needed. These act locally in the lungs or centrally in the brain. Such drugs used include.

Local action

(1) Expectorants. Drugs that stimulate the cough and make it more effective by increasing the lungs' secretions. They may or may not help.
(2) Mucolytics. Drugs that reduce the stickiness of the lung secretions. The commonest is bromhexine (Bisolvon is the trade name). One or two tablets can be taken 3 times a day and there is a liquid form.
(3) Decongestants. There are a great number of these often combining a decongestant (usually ephedrine) with an

antihistamine and codeine. Commonly used are actified compound linctus and phensedyl cough linctus and they often seem to help patients.

Central action

The commonest drugs, in increasing strength, are:

(1) Codeine linctus.
(2) Pholcodeine linctus.
(3) Methadone linctus.
(4) Diamorphine linctus.

They all act as cough suppressants.

It is often best to combine two drugs acting in different ways, e.g. a mucolytic (Bromhexine) and codeine linctus.

URINARY INCONTINENCE

This is rather a common and distressing symptom in severely ill patients and there are several reasons why it happens.

- Urinary infections. These are common and cause increased frequency of urination and pain on passing urine as well as occasional incontinence. Treatment is with an antibiotic.
- Cancer in the pelvis, irritating or pressing on the bladder can cause increased frequency of passing urine and occasionally incontinence. Treatment is designed to shrink the tumour (surgery, radiotherapy, or chemotherapy). Treatment with radiation to the bladder can cause scarring and shrinkage and a drug, cyclophosphamide, can cause irritation of the bladder (Appendix A).
- Interference with nerves to the bladder. Occasionally cancer can press on the spinal cord and interfere with the way the bladder functions. This is usually accompanied with weakness of the legs and loss or altered sensation in the lower half of the body. *Immediate* radiotherapy or surgery to remove the pressure on the spinal cord should always be arranged in all but the most ill patients. If this condition is not treated urgently paralysis of the legs and permanent incontinence will develop. Any patient with weakness of their legs, loss, or changed sensation, or incontinence should get the advice of their doctor quickly.

- Passing increased quantities of urine (polyuria). This is often due to diabetes which is treated in the usual way. Kidney failure can also cause this problem and is also treated in the normal way.

CATHETERIZATION

If incontinence cannot be controlled easily then a thin tube (catheter) is passed into the bladder. This should be done in a sterile manner and the catheter is kept in place by a small balloon which is inflated when the catheter is in the bladder; this is painless. If a catheter is needed over a long period then it should be changed regularly (about once a month) and each change of catheter covered by two days' antibiotics to prevent the introduction of bacteria into the bladder.

The use of a catheter is extremely important if there is persistent incontinence. It is very important to avoid leakage of urine as this may result in infection, sores and ulcers, making life miserable. Often, quite wrongly, catheterization is unnecessarily delayed.

URINARY RETENTION (the inability to pass urine)

This is less common but usually requires catheterization until the cause can be taken away (for example an operation for an enlarged prostate).

LACK OF SLEEP (Insomnia)

Many patients who are severely ill suffer from insomnia because of pain, anxiety, frequency of urination, and shortness of breath. If lack of sleep is due to depression then specific treatment (page 309) is needed. Pain should be treated (page 294), with adequate regular doses of pain-killers. Urinary frequency should be treated as above. If sedatives are needed to help a patient to sleep the best drugs are those falling into a group called benzodiazepins. The best known of these is diazepam (Valium is the trade name) and another, nitrazepam (Mogadon) is also commonly used. The dose is 5–10 mg taken at night. Elderly patients who become confused by these drugs may be better off with chloral (trade name— Welldorm) or chlormethiazole (Hemineverin). Temazepam is a useful drug as its break-down products are not active. For those who are awakened by severe sweating (common in some types of cancer) indomethanin (Indocid) tablets can be helpful.

DEPRESSION

Everybody with cancer will suffer some degree of depression. It is the normal response to learning the diagnosis and is common during treatment. This 'reactive' depression responds best to sympathetic discussion but some people become emotionally exhausted by months of worry may gradually become apathetic and it is this apathy that can quickly turn to real depression. Depression removes the will to recover and needs urgent treatment.

Modern anti-depressant tablets, given as a single dose at night—the commonest are called tricyclics—can do much to help lift mood and this gives the patient an opportunity to discuss worries with a skilled therapist or doctor. Treatment for pain or any worrying symptom must not be ignored as this may do much to relieve depression. Depression is often coupled with anxiety and this is discussed below.

ANXIETY

Anxiety is characterized by a collection of unpleasant nervous symptoms and is the body's response to excess stress and tension. Once this is seen as the problem it is important for the patient to realize that these feelings are of no medical significance whatsoever, though it is all very bewildering and distressing. It may be caused by worry about:

- Curability.
- Fear of treatment.
- Fear of being in hospital.
- Fear of future symptoms.
- Financial worries.
- Worries about outpatient visits.
- Worries about spouse and children.
- Spiritual worries.

Apart from the constant feelings of tension, other physical symptoms occur in 'attacks' — panic spasms, palpitations, chest pain, giddiness, nausea, trembling spells, inability to take a deep breath, as well as depression and sleeplessness.

It is important for a doctor to take time to talk to and listen to the fears of anyone who is anxious and this is often more useful than drugs. Drugs (diazepam) may be useful initially to help settle the symptoms but regular discussion with a doctor will keep problems in perspective and eventually help to calm the patient down. A clear explanation of the symptoms themselves and that the cause is emotional rather than physical is most important to anyone suffering from anxiety and this explanation itself can help the patient to find peace of mind. Emotional problems are almost more upsetting than physical distress for relatives but can often be helped by sympathetic care.

RESTLESSNESS AND CONFUSION

It is very upsetting when a close relative eventually fails to recognize anyone, becomes disorientated, noisy, and restless. Sometimes it is caused by drugs and a dose adjustment will help but often the cause is not easy to find. Confused patients are greatly helped by seeing familiar faces and being (if possible) in their own surroundings. Restlessness or aggressive confusion can be helped by drugs such as chlorpromazine.

CARE OF ULCERATING CANCERS

A minority of cancers grow so that they affect the skin and become ulcerated. This is particularly distressing as the cancer is now visible or may even smell. If possible, treatment with radiotherapy or chemotherapy should be used to reduce the tumour. It occurs most commonly in cancer of the breast and disfigurement of this sort is particularly difficult for women — especially scrupulously clean women to bear. They often isolate themselves and many become distressed thinking that they smell.

- If there is infection a seven-day course of a broad spectrum antibiotic should be given. This reduces infection and any unpleasant smell.
- The ulcerated area should be cleaned often 2 or 3 times a day. Eusol diluted half and half with water is very helpful though this may be uncomfortable in sensitive areas. Betadine and Hibitane (trade names) are alternative antiseptics that do not sting. If the area is ulcerated and wet then eusol (50 per cent) with paraffin (50 per cent) can be applied to the area using gauze soaked in the solution. If the area is dry it can be cleaned with a

salt solution (saline) and a dry dressing applied. Gentian violet
is often very effective for drying moist ulcers.

- If there is bleeding from the ulcer (especially from where it
sticks to a dressing) a special non-adhesive dressing should be
used. Sometimes radiotherapy can be useful. There is seldom
need to fear a sudden haemorrhage, as many patients do.

With careful dressing and care, often by a visiting nurse, the
problems of a large ulcerated area can be minimized.

CHAPTER NINETEEN

Talking about cancer
with Susan Williams

Cancer is the disease people dread most. It is a subject fraught with myth, mystery, and most of all silence. It is usually assumed that all cancers are painful and fatal; a disease for which there is 'no cure' and 'no hope'. However, there has been much progress in the control of cancer, and this is not widely understood.

There is a gradual awareness amongst those looking after cancer patients, led by cancer sufferers, that an honest approach to the situation is the most sensible and right policy and it is assumed that anyone wishing to read this book will be seeking truthful information, however sad it may sometimes seem.

After a cancer has been found a decision must be made whether the patient should be told. In the past doctors have talked around the diagnosis using words such as 'ulcers', 'cysts', 'lesions', etc., but in the past ten years it has become more usual to discuss the diagnosis openly with the patient and people do indeed find it easier to deal with the disease and its treatment if they understand exactly what is going on. For most it is just the confirmation of what they had strongly suspected. In situations where the patient is not told but only close family are given the diagnosis this can be very destructive: the patient becomes isolated and the family lie. Usually the patient is aware of their cancer, but cannot discuss it with their husband or wife in case of causing distress, whilst the spouse knows too but is also frightened of talking about it, causing imaginable tension between the couple.

For most patients a simple knowledge of the disease and its treatment is helpful and any questions they have should be answered with honesty tempered with sensitivity. This book should be of great factual help but is only intended as a back-up to normal communication between the patient and those looking after him and it cannot be stressed too strongly that good communication is very important. Every patient should try to find someone with whom they can easily discuss their treatment, fears and worries, be it the family doctor, a nurse, or a good friend. Such discussions with medical staff, including an under-standing of tests, treatment, and prognosis and what it means for each individual patient must be carefully planned and should proceed at a pace the patient can handle comfortably. If the patient is allowed to lead the discussion the correct pace is assured. A good proportion of this book deals with how and why the patient is treated but every hospital has its own way of doing things, and it is useful to ask about the treatment and investigations that are being planned for you. Some hospitals prepare a short leaflet outlining the treatment and its side-effects asking the patient to get in contact if they have problems.

Surprisingly little research has been done about emotional reactions to cancer even though difficulties caused by poor communication, treatment, pain, and changes in role or life style are very common. These problems usually parallel the three different stages of the disease (remember many patients do **not** have advancing disease). The initial phase at the time cancer is detected and diagnosed. Intermediate phase, when treatment is underway, but the outcome for success or failure is uncertain and for some an advancing phase when, treatment has failed to control the tumour, and death must be faced.

DETECTION

The discovery of a strange lump or persistent symptom that doesn't go away on its own is often as shocking as learning for the first time that it is indeed cancer. The apparent gravity of the diagnosis may be compounded by the doctor's silence, his uncomfortable 'small talk', serious manner, or vain reassurance. Often the patient is afraid to ask what is wrong, and so a conspiracy of silence develops.

The next period is one of waiting for the outcome of the exhaustive tests and biopsies which follow the initial examination. This is a trying time, and it is particularly important that the patient feels involved in the tests, knows why they are being performed and what they will eventually show. Patients must *ask* about the results if they want to know about them.

WHEN CANCER IS DIAGNOSED

When the diagnosis has been made and confirmed by the doctor an open and friendly talk with both patient and relatives, about the treatment involved and possible outlook, undertaken in an optimistic a way as the facts allow is valuable for all concerned. It clears the air and opens the path for questions and frank discussion of fears and feelings; but all too often this does not happen, the patient becomes visibly withdrawn and depressed or is tearful and those around then try to ignore what is happening and a tense situation builds up. Some people are very open and composed about their illness and are keen to discuss it but again those around find such free expression of a 'taboo' subject uncomfortable. Perhaps it is most sensible to find a wise counsellor, preferably a doctor or any experienced friend, who can view problems from a detached point of view. Though a platitude, 'a trouble shared is a trouble halved' is often very true for the cancer patient.

Coping with death

Coming to terms with dying is very difficult for anyone to imagine and will require skilled counselling. Anger, fear and bitterness at the situation, are all emotions that need exploring.

It seems, to the patient, that those who care little for life live to an old age, whilst those to revel in its challenges are stricken with illness prematurely. Anger soon follows, caused by the threat of death, and is then followed by a painful sense of bitterness which is often not recognized by others.

In their effort to help the patient repress unpleasant emotions and sometimes to defend themselves against anxiety, others, make it hard for the patient to express feelings. Communication is further hampered by the patient's own guilt over the anger they feel and depression soon follows and family and friends, taking their cue from the patient, leave them alone or become anxious or irritated — and a communication stalemate results. Often visitors are tense and ill at ease and this leads to the patient making cheery conversation about everything but their real feelings. The feelings of bitterness are, therefore, not readily got rid of. Sadness, tears, and helplessness are easily understood and result in empathy for the patient; bitterness does not and the patient quickly learns this and tries to avoid expressing it.

Patients can be helped by:

- Emphasizing that denial and anger can be useful if expressed.
- Encouraging them to grumble. Self-pity in small doses helps a lot.
- Making them realize their feelings are respectable so that they don't feel guilty.
- Discussion of feelings is often best *not* done with relatives who are too involved.
- Tell them it is not wicked to hate doctors, family or God.
- Get them to vent their feelings — 'kicking the cat' is healthy.
- Above all talk to them realistically. Some think this means pessimism but for many patients it means optimism. The dying have a great freedom — nothing more can happen to them so they can do what they want and become great risk takers. The rest of us are too afraid of risks which stifles life.
- Guilt should be assuaged.

CONTINUING PROBLEMS

- No matter how great the patient's optimism there is always an awareness that cancer *might* return. Although with time this lessens, it is nonetheless there. They cannot be completely reassured and this may eventually make family and friends angry with them. Patients having a check-up years after their cancer was treated may feel anxious and unwell for several days before seeing their doctor; no-one emerges from the experience as if it had never happened, like all bad experiences.
- Treatment, especially surgery, may disfigure and this is especially important with certain operations such as mastectomy. For weeks after such an operation patients often won't look at their scar, feel lopsided, as though they have lost their femininity and are unattractive. They hate how they look and feel depressed and over-react to any new loss. Dressing and undressing are a painful reminder of the loss and wearing some clothes becomes unthinkable despite assurance that a posthesis would make her look a normal woman.
- Pain is depressing, frightening, and tiring and is very difficult to describe. Because of this it is important that every effort is made to control any pain (page 293).
- Open communication cannot resolve all the problems but for most patients it certainly helps. Empathetic support from all concerned makes the unbearable, possible to bear, and many

who think that they will never cope often show great strength and resilience which surprises even themselves. Ask much of patients and it is seldom that one is disappointed in their fortitude and cheerfulness.

DYING

Most of this book is concerned with the active treatment of cancer and the enormous advances that have occurred in the past 10–20 years. Unfortunately some patients die from their tumour. They are often told that nothing more can be done for them: this is seldom if ever true.

Methods for controlling a patient's individual symptoms (Chapter Sixteen) continue to get better and 'active' treatment to improve the quality of a patient's life becomes as important as earlier treatments that attempted to 'cure' the patient. Unfortunately, all too often the transition from attempts to cure cancer to treatment for symptoms only is made arbitrarily and suddenly. It has been said that the dying (or terminal) phase of a disease can be defined as beginning at the moment the doctor says 'Nothing more can be done' and then withdraws from the patient. What he really means is that there is nothing more surgically to be done (if he is a surgeon) or no radiotherapy will help (if he is a radiotherapist). The same is true for all other specialists.

Because communication has often been poor earlier in the disease it may be impossible for the patient to help make decisions regarding further therapy. If patients are to make known their feelings about their management this can only be achieved by prolonged discussion of the physical and social consequences of treatment. If this does not happen then some patients will insist on 'everything being tried' or respond with 'do not let them do anything' whilst others with a mistaken bravado will ask 'to be experimented on'. A rational decision is very difficult and patients should never be asked to make decisions by themselves. It is the physician's job to explore the possibilities and then to arrive at a conclusion which he then puts to the patient and often the family for final ratification. Occasionally two treatments will have equal merit. If the effects on the patient differ he must be allowed to decide with guidance, which to choose. We all like to be involved with our own destiny and nothing generates a better relationship between patient and doctor.

If a decision is made to stop 'curative' treatment it is imperative that the patient does not feel abandoned. Doctors often (because of their impotence and sense of failure) feel threatened by a dying patient and respond by gradually ignoring them, but this is when the patient needs the greatest time and skill from their doctor. The increasing number of hospices (also called continuing care units) emphasizes the general lack of these skills that still exists. Continuing care units are not special places for the dying; they are as the name implies, units concerned with improving the quality of life of the cancer patient. They have expertise in the treatment of symptoms and relief of physical and mental distress that allows the patient to concentrate on living as full a life as possible. The aim of most hospices is to get patients home to their family and friends and most have a team of specialist doctors and nurses who will support the patient at home in any way they can.

The patient

A person who has suffered surgical treatment that caused loss of part of the body needs to spend adequate time getting over or mourning this loss. Patients whose families, friends, and doctors are made uncomfortable by this may need professional counselling. Patients who despite such support remain unable to discuss their illness and treatment realistically may be going through a stage of denial. If this is prolonged they may need similar help. The longer this process of adjustment is delayed the greater is the likelihood of depression. An essential part of mourning is the continuous testing of reality and a final painful recognition of the loss is essential if the patient is to come to terms with their illness. This process takes time but surprisingly patients adjust to loss much more effectively than do most relatives.

Similar reactions occur with radiotherapy and chemotherapy and patients should expect that feelings of depression, anger (often irrational anger or irritability), bitterness, sadness, and deep disappointment will occur and they should be reassured that these are quite normal reactions to all that is happening to

318

them. Patients often prefer to be with close relatives and friends during this time to obtain mutual support.

Family and friends

To the family and close friends a cancer patient is someone who is probably suffering physical and mental pain. Family and friends are shocked; they feel helpless, not knowing what to say or how to express the things they want to say. They may suddenly be faced with the possibility of death, loss of a loved one and wonder how to prepare for this without showing the patient what they dread to admit to themselves. Whilst they are feeling these things the patient struggles with how he has let them down and frantically wishes he could wave a magic wand to change the reality of these terrible events. They wonder if family and friends will be able to stay with them through all this, but cannot ask for fear that they won't be understood or will upset their relatives by fearfulness and excessive dependency. Most patients need to be 'forgiven' for their illness; any severe illness places added burdens on those around the patient and they are aware of this. They also need to be reassured that their cancer is not a punishment for past misdeeds.

Advice to helpers

A relative, friend, or doctor who wants to help a patient must let them know that they are not going to desert them and that they are trying to understand some of the struggles the patient is experiencing. Someone to whom they can talk as little or as much as they want without embarrassment is often the best support. Patience and an ability to *listen* rather than to give advice is usually best. Tell the patient of your optimisim and hope (if this is appropriate) but be serious and realistic, never maudlin or pessimistic. Go with the patient if you can, to check-ups, radiotheraphy, chemotheraphy, or any hospital visits. Show pleasure with any progress but do not try to push him back to health. Daily expressions of 'you do look better today' when the patient is getting worse are stupid and can only cause frustration, anger, and resentment. It is hard to resist the temptation, but don't do it. Be aware that the patient may have ups and downs, will have inexplicable period of irritability, depression, and dependency. This is difficult for friends and relatives and they themselves must be able to let off steam with others and may often need advice from their family doctor or friends.

Families and friends must, above all, remember that the patient needs to mourn. They must allow the patient time to grieve accepting that it is a normal, healthy process which they must pass painfully through in order to get successfully over their loss and to resolve their normal depression. As mentioned before patients do it much better than relatives — even if their emotional reactions may appear more dramatic.

In the hospital

Communication with doctors is particularly difficult and most patients feel more comfortable with and talk more openly to nurses. Doctors can give too much hope or cause too much fear for the relationship to be easy. In addition the doctor plays out his role together with the patient and this traditional role has put obligations, which may suppress open discussion, on both. If there is hope, then it is best that it is given quickly and clearly to the patient. Most patients feel too frightened to ask threatening questions and use many devices, such as telling themselves, 'I'll wait till I'm stronger', to avoid asking. It is easy for a doctor to discourage questions by his attitude; this may be excessively reassuring or defensive. Some doctors may even seem to criticize a lack of questions but it is best for the patient to make the pace, they should be given every opportunity to question but never have unwanted information forced on them. The doctor-patient relationship is complicated by each other's perception of the cancer and their response to it. The patient may in some way sense that they have disappointed or failed their doctor by having such an onerous disease or by failing treatment. They may feel that the physician would rather not see them because there is no 'cure' and this is compounded by the doctor's feeling of inadequacy and failure in the face of a difficult or even insoluble problem.

Patients with advancing cancer, in addition to sympathetic and skilled psychological support, need expert treatment to control symptoms. Some of the methods of treatment used are described in Chapter Eighteen and it is very important that care is taken to ensure that every measure is used to control physical problems. This may frequently be done by hospital doctors working together with the patient's GP but sometimes it is useful for the patient to have the help of a team of doctors or nurses from a continuing care centre.

CHAPTER TWENTY

What are trials?

Improvements in the treatment of cancer can only come from knowing more about what makes tumours grow and from new techniques of surgery, radiotherapy, and chemotherapy. All new types of treatment have eventually to be tested in people and rather than allow haphazard use of new treatment on different patients most hospitals will test the treatment in a trial (sometimes called a study).

Why do we need trials?

Although there have been improvements in cancer care during the past fifty years we still need better treatments with fewer side-effects. Scientists are continually devising new ways of treating cancer and a small number of these treatments, which appear promising, are tested in patients. Doctors are also looking for different ways of using the treatments that we already have and the only way to find out if any of these new treatments work is to treat a group of patients, and to see how they fare, in other words to run a trial.

What, exactly, is a trial?

In a trial doctors pick out a group of patients they will treat; this means they will choose a particular tumour, only include patients in a certain age range or stage. This group of patients will be given the new treatment and are carefully watched.

Trials may be of two basic types. If only one treatment is tested then all patients may be treated in the same way. Alternatively the new treatment may be compared directly with another treatment. The other treatment may be the conventional way of treating the tumour or may even be no treatment at all, if no useful treatment is available. The aim of a trial of the two treatments is to compare their usefulness directly. In this type of trial it is common to choose the treatment of each patient by chance (randomization).

This means that the doctor and patient do not know which treatment is to be given until the patient agrees to the trial. Obviously, in these circumstances both types of treatment must be fully discussed and be acceptable to both the patient and doctor.

ARE THERE ANY SAFEGUARDS FOR PATIENTS?

Recently the concept of 'informed consent' has become accepted. Informed consent means that the patient has been given information and understands all about their disease and its possible treatments and their side-effects, so that they can make a rational decision about entering a trial. In addition to discussion of the patient's disease and the trial, doctors in the United States are obliged by law to get patients to sign a form giving consent to the trial. This form sets out all the facts about the treatment; some hospitals in Europe have similar documents though many do not require consent by signature.

Any patient agreeing to go into a trial must do so voluntarily and should know that the treatment is new or 'experimental'. The doctor should explain the treatment and answer all questions and give the patient time to think about it. Patients always have the right to refuse to enter a study or may discontinue it at any time and this should not affect the patient's care in any way. All trials in a hospital have to be approved by an 'ethical committee'. This mixed group of doctors, scientists, and lay people have the job of making sure that any trial is sensible, well designed, and is ethical. As well as any possible benefit from the treatment being tested, patients may gain from the extra attention that they may receive because of the trial.

Patients faced with the possibility of being tested in a trial should ask all the questions they need to help decide if this is what they want. Suggested questions are included in Chapters Twelve, Thirteen, Fourteen on surgery, radiotherapy, and chemotherapy. General questions you may want to ask about the new treatment include:

- What are the possible benefits?
- What are the risks?
- What is known about the treatment?
- Will the new treatment be compared with another treatment?
- If so, will I be able to choose the treatment I want or will this be chosen by chance?

- How good are other treatments?
- What are the side-effects of other treatments
- How long will the trial go on for?
- Will I need to be in hospital for the new treatment?
- Do I need to come into hospital for alternative treatments?
- How often is the new treatment given?

WHAT TYPES OF TRIALS ARE THERE?

Most trials of new treatments test anticancer drugs though similar trials are used to test other treatments. When a new drug is available for testing in patients it goes through a series of trials.

(1) Phase 1 trial

This is the first time a drug is used in people and the aim is to find out its side-effects and to select the best dose. These trials are only done in a few special cancer centres and in patients for whom there is no known effective treatment. Drugs in phase 1 trials are given in low doses at first and the dose gradually increased till there are severe side-effects. As the drug has never been used in man unexpected side-effects are not uncommon and occasionally patients may die from side-effects. Phase 1 trials are therefore hazardous for the patient and the chance of any benefit is small. Patients receiving new drugs in a phase 1 trial should not expect miracles, the most they should expect is that the trial may eventually help others.

Despite the problems of phase 1 studies there is no way round the need to test new drugs in human trials. Most patients should not consider entering these studies, though some may do so in special centres as it offers a small hope and is a way of helping others with cancer. These trials never compare two treatments and the treatment is not randomized (chosen by chance).

(2) Phase 2 trials

At this stage the doctor knows what the safe dose is and most of the side-effects of the new drug. The main effort of a phase 2 trial is to try to find out how effective an anticancer drug it is. Because we don't know if the drug will work it is only ethical if the patients chosen are those no longer responding to the usual treatments or those who have a tumour for which there is no useful treatment.

The chances of benefit from a new phase 2 drug are poor but every few years a new drug comes along that is very active and patients may then gain from the trial. These drugs are experimental and are not available except in trials so that patients who are anxious to be treated with a new drug can only do so if they accept a trial. Most phase 2 trials do not compare treatments and are not randomized.

(3) Phase 3 trials

Only drugs shown to be effective in phase 2 trials are tested in this phase. The drug may be used alone or together with other drugs in a combination. Either way the new treatments are often compared with another treatment and randomized trials (choice of treatment by chance) are common. Because the treatment has been shown to work, the chances of success are good though it may be no better than currently available treatments; this can only be shown by the trial.

(4) Trials of adjuvant therapy

This is the use of treatment after the patient has undergone an initial operation (or other treatment) that may have cured the cancer. Because there is still a risk of the cancer growing back, even though all the visible tumour has been removed, it is worth seeing if additional treatment will prevent this. Chemotherapy is usually used and most experience of adjuvant therapy has been gained in breast cancer (page 143).

Not all patients will have their disease grow back but it is not possible to predict those that will. If treatment, as we think it does, works best when there is least tumour then the greatest chance of cure for those who will relapse is adjuvant therapy when there is no visible disease. However, in addition to this possible advantage all patients receiving adjuvant treatment will have marked side-effects. In order to learn if adjuvant therapy is beneficial trials have divided patients, by chance, into two groups: those who receive adjuvant treatment and a group who have no further treatment. Patients need to know if they are to be entered into such a trial as the treatments that may be chosen are very different and they should consider if it is a good thing for them to enter the trial. Trials testing adjuvant treatment are very important and there is a fine balance between advantage and disadvantage for patients. If patients can accept the necessity for selecting the treatment by chance then it is reasonabe to consider accepting an adjuvant trial. It is too early to say, from the trials that are running, if this approach works. Adjuvant trials need large numbers and have to run for 5–10 years.

Some patients are worried that they will be used as guinea pigs to experiment on: they need not worry. Although trials are scientific experiments testing new treatments the very fact that this is being done in a trial, and not haphazardously, means that the treatment is carefully controlled. Ethical committees ensure that the trial is sensibly conducted and fair to the patient. Patients should always feel free to opt out of a trial and no pressure should be exerted to try to persuade patients into a trial. Good trials often benefit patients though in phase 1 and 2 studies no benefit should be expected.

CHAPTER TWENTY-ONE

Ostomies: colostomies, ileostomies, and urinary diversions

An ostomy is a surgical operation to make a new pathway for the discharge of the body's wastes; the opening on to the surface of skin is known as a stoma. These operations are done for a number of diseases of the bowel and urinary tract including cancer.

When the new opening is formed from the colon the stoma is called a colostomy and when it is formed from the ileum (part of the small bowel) the stoma is known as an ileostomy. Both these stomas discharge faeces, but the one chosen will depend on where the cancer is.

In cancer of the bladder it may be necessary to totally remove the bladder and the ureters (tubes that connect the kidneys and bladder) may be brought directly up to the skin or may be connected to the ileum (part of the small bowel) which is brought up to the skin as a stoma (this is called an ileal conduit).

After an ostomy operation the patient will lose voluntary control over the discharge of the wastes concerned and they have to wear a special appliance for the collection of this waste. Despite this, there is no reason why a patient with a stoma should not live a perfectly normal life: family, social, business, and sporting. However, adjustment is difficult and patients need help in learning to live with their ostomy. Some find it difficult to manage the appliance, but even if this is no problem they may find it impossible to resume a normal social life. Help from special stoma nurses and ostomy associations is available even before an operation is done and it is well worth patients contacting local associations. Members of these groups usually have an ostomy themselves and can give practical help and encouragement from their own experience. Although many colostomies are permanent some may be temporary and these are usually done when an operation has relieved a bowel obstruction. A temporary colostomy may be removed after several months and the normal bowel joined together again.

COLOSTOMIES

A colostomy is *sigmoid, descending, transverse,* or *ascending* depending on which part of the colon is used to make the stoma (Figure 45). If properly cared for and fitted the appliance can be completely odourless and invisible to others.

Descending and sigmoid colostomies

This is usually a permanent operation and is most commonly done when it is impossible to remove a cancer that is low down in the bowel without causing incontinence. The remaining part of the colon still absorbs water and because of this semisolid stool will probably be formed.

Some patients may eventually have motions at more or less regular times during the day and can manage without a bag for part of the day (a stoma cap is adequate). Irrigation or enemas can be used to regulate the colostomy to prevent 'unscheduled' movements though this should only be done on a doctor's advice.

Transverse colostomy

This is often a temporary colostomy. The nature of discharge is unpredictable though it is usually semi-liquid and a stoma appliance is usually worn continuously. As the discharge contains digestive enzymes the appliance used must protect the skin around the stoma and special seals are used.

Ascending colon

The discharge is liquid and flows almost continuously. Because it contains digestive enzymes protection of the skin around the stoma is important. It is usually looked after in the same way as an ileostomy (see below) and a special seal is needed around the stoma.

328

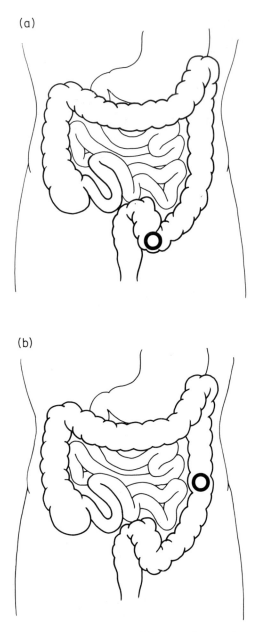

(a)

(b)

Figure 45 Diagrammatic representation of the large bowel showing the different positions where a stoma may be placed. (a) sigmoid colostomy, (b) descending colostomy, (c) transverse colostomy, (d) ascending colostomy

(c)

(d)

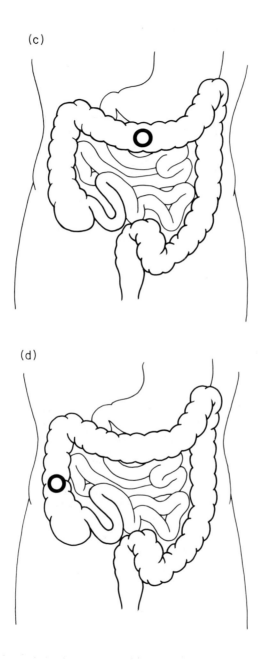

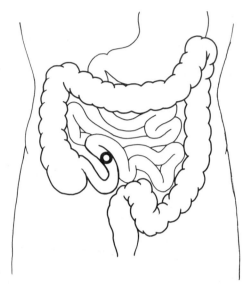

Figure 46 Diagrammatic representation of the position of an ileostomy stoma

ILEOSTOMY

This ostomy is made using the ileum, the part of the small intestine farthest from the stomach (Figure 46). An ileostomy is usually performed using the last part of the ileum just before the colon and is done when the whole of the colon and rectum is removed (see page 13).

As there is no longer a colon to absorb water and form solid stools the ileostomy discharges liquid which flows almost continuously. This contains digestive enzymes and the ileostomy stoma is made to protrude up to an inch into the appliance so that the skin is protected. This is very important because the enzymes will digest the skin and cause the appliance to leak which in turn worsens the problem.

After operations requiring an ileostomy the aim must be total rehabilitation. Skin protection is basic and a properly fitted appliance is essential. An ideal appliance should be simple to put in, provide a leak-proof seal, and be odourless. Because they change in size and shape the stoma should be remeasured periodically and the appliance changed as required.

ILEAL CONDUIT

This operation is so-called because the surgeon converts a segment of the ileum (about 15 cm) into a pipe, or conduit, for urinary drainage. The ureters are disconnected from the bladder (which is usually removed) and are joined to one end of the ileum, the other end of the ileum being brought through the abdominal wall to form a stoma. The segment of ileum removed from the small intestine survives on its own blood supply and the rest of the bowel is rejoined and continues to work normally.

There is no 'voluntary' control of the stoma which discharges a drop of urine every 10–20 seconds. A urostomy bag is worn over the stoma and should be leak-proof, easily fitted, odourless, and have the facility for night drainage.

Details on the use of ostomy appliances can be obtained from the various associations and groups included in Appendix D. Patients with an ostomy can, in the United Kingdom, apply for a certificate of exemption from prescription charges for equipment available under the National Health Service.

PATIENT NOTES

Doctor's name:

    Surgeon: Telephone:

    Radiotherapist: Telephone:

    Medical oncologist: Telephone:

    Family practitioner: Telephone:

    Other doctors: Telephone:

Nurse's name:

    Chemotherapy nurse: Telephone:

    Mastectomy or ostomy nurse: Telephone:

    Other nurses: Telephone:

Hospital: Telephone:

Ward: Telephone:

PATIENT NOTES

Questions:

Answers:

PATIENT NOTES

Treatment regime:

PATIENT NOTES

Appointments:

PATIENT NOTES

Additional information:

Drugs commonly used to treat cancer

Drug	Method by which it is given	Common side-effects (those in capitals are commonly troublesome)
Alkylating agents. A large group of drugs that react chemically with DNA (the genetic material in a cell controlling its division and function)		
BCNU	Into a vein	NAUSEA and VOMITING, RISK OF INFECTION OR BRUISING and BLEEDING, pain at site of injection, infertility.
Busulphan	By mouth	RISK OF INFECTION or BRUISING and BLEEDING, infertility, skin pigmentation.
CCNU	By mouth	NAUSEA AND VOMITING, risk of infection and bruising and bleeding, infertility.
Chlorambucil	By mouth	Risk of infection and bruising and bleeding, infertility.
Chlorozotocin	Into a vein	Risk of infection and bruising and bleeding, nausea and vomiting, infertility.
Cis platin	Into a vein	NAUSEA AND VOMITING, risk of infection and bruising and bleeding, kidney damage if not given carefully with fluids, hearing loss for high toncs, diarrhoea.
Cyclophosphamide	Into a vein or by mouth	Nausea and vomiting, bladder irritation (cystitis), sterility, loss of hair, sore mouth, risk of infection or bruising and bleeding.
DTIC	Into a vein	Risk of infection or bruising and bleeding, NAUSEA AND VOMITING, pain at injection site, temperature, infertility.

337

Drug	Method by which it is given	Common side-effects (those in capitals are commonly troublesome)
Mephalan	By mouth	Risk of infection or bruising and bleeding, infertility.
Methyl CCNU	By mouth	Risk of infection or bruising and bleeding, NAUSEA AND VOMITING, infertility.
Mustine	Into·a vein	NAUSEA AND VOMITING, pain at site of injection, risk of infection or bruising or bleeding, HAIR LOSS.
Streptozotocin	Into a vein	Risk of infection or bruising and bleeding, nausea and vomiting, pain at injection site.
Thiotepa	Into a vein	Risk of infection or bruising and bleeding, nausea and vomiting, infertility.

Antibiotic group. A group of drugs each of which is produced by different strains of bacteria. However, they only have a very weak effect against bacterial but can kill tumour cells.

Drug	Method by which it is given	Common side-effects
Actinomycin D	Into a vein	NAUSEA AND VOMITING, risk of infection or bruising and bleeding, pain at injection site, sore mouth.
Adriamycin	Into a vein	Nausea and vomiting, risk of infection or bruising and bleeding, pain at injection site, heart damage if an *excessive* total dose is given, COMPLETE HAIR LOSS.
Bleomycin	Into a vein, under the skin by injection, into a muscle by injection	Temperature and shivering, skin pigmentation and thickening, lung damage if an excessive total dose is given, hair loss.
Daunorubicin	Into a vein	Nausea and vomiting, risk of infection or bruising and bleeding, pain at injection site, heart damage if *excessive* total dose is given, COMPLETE HAIR LOSS.
Mithramycin	Into a vein	Risk of infection or bruising and bleeding, temperature, pain at injection site.
Mitomycin C	Into a vein	Risk of infection or bruising and bleeding, pain at injection site, nausea and vomiting, hair loss.

Drug	Method by which it is given	Common side-effects (those in capitals are commonly troublesome)
Antimetabolites. Drugs that interfere with DNA production.		
Cytosine arabinoside	Into a vein	Risk of infection, bruising or bleeding, sore mouth.
5-Fluorouracil	Into a vein, occasionally by mouth	Risk of infection, bruising or bleeding, nausea and vomiting, sore mouth, hair loss.
6-Mercaptopurine	By mouth	Risk of infection, bruising and bleeding.
Methotrexate	Into a vein or by mouth	Risk of infection, bruising or bleeding, sore mouth, kidney damage when in high doses.
Mitotic inhibitors. Drugs that interfere directly with cell division.		
Vinblastine	Into a vein	Risk of infection or bruising and bleeding, pain at site of injection, numbness and tingling of hands and feet.
Vincristine	Into a vein	NUMBNESS AND TINGLING OF HANDS AND FEET, pain at site of injection, loss of hair.
Vindesine	Into a vein	Risk of infection or bruising and bleeding, NUMBNESS AND TINGLING OF HANDS AND FEET, pain at injection site, loss of hair.
Miscellaneous. Drugs working in various ways not included in the preceding main groups.		
Asparaginase	Into a vein	ALLERGIC REACTIONS, TEMPERATURE, sleepiness, high blood sugar.
Etoposide	Into a vein, by mouth	Risk of infection or bruising and bleeding, LOSS OF HAIR, nausea and vomiting.
Hexamethylmelamine	By mouth	NAUSEA AND VOMITING, risk of infection or bruising and bleeding.
Hydroxyurea	By mouth	Risk of infection or bruising and bleeding, nausea and vomiting.

Diets

As a general principle patients with a poor appetite should eat small regular meals or snacks and should avoid trying to eat large 'normal' meals. Their diet should contain both protein and plenty of calories (energy). Important foods which can be prepared many different ways include:

cheese	yoghurt
cottage cheese	ice-cream
milk or cream	nuts and peanut butter
powdered milk	meat and fish
eggs	peas and beans

For most patients 'small and often' is best. It is not always possible for patients to eat a balanced diet and special liquid food supplements (page 300) and vitamins may be helpful.

Special diets may be prescribed for particular situations such as after an operation or during radiotherapy. These include the following.

Clear liquid diet. Used when there is severe intolerance of food especially soon after an operation or during severe nausea and vomiting.

	Allowed	Forbidden
Drinks	Fizzy drinks, decaffeinated coffee, fruit drinks, tea, and water	Milk or milk drinks
Cheese	None	All
Desserts	Jellies, sorbet	All others
Eggs	None	All
Fats	None	All
Fruit juices	Apple, grape, strained citrus, and cranberry	All others
Fish and meat	None	All
Milk	None	All
Potatoes, rice and pasta	None	All
Soup	Clear fat-free broths, con- sommé and bouillon	All others
Vegetable	Tomato juice, strained vegetable broth	All others
Condiments and spices	Salt	All others
Sweets	Honey, syrups	All others

Full liquid diet. Used when a person is acutely ill and is unable to chew or swallow solid food. Includes foods that are liquid at room temperature and is useful for patients with a severe sore mouth.

	Allowed	Forbidden
Drinks	All	None
Bread and cereal	Refined or strained cereals for gruel or porridge	solid breads
Cheese	In soups	All others
Desserts	Jelly, junket, baked custard, sorbets, ice-cream, yoghurt	All others
Eggs	Egg nog	Fried, scrambled, hard boiled
Fats	Butter, cream, oils, margerine	All others
Fruit juices	Citrus fruit juices, strained fruit juices, all other juices, thin purée of fruit	All others
Fish and meat	Small quantities of puréed fish or meat in broth	All others
Milk	Milk and flavoured milks, ice-cream, milk shakes, plain yoghurt	All others
Potatoes, rice, and pasta	Puréed potato in soups	All others
Vegetable	Puréed vegetables for soups, vegetable juices	All others
Condiments and spices	Salt, flavouring extracts	All others
Sweets	Honey, syrups	All others

Soft diet. A transition between a liquid diet and a normal diet. Useful when patients have a sore mouth or difficulty in swallowing. Foods may be made soft by cooking, mashing, or puréeing.

	Allowed	*Forbidden*
Drinks	All	None
Bread and cereal	All except —	Bread and biscuits containing seeds, nuts, fruits, whole-meal breads, and bran
Flour	All except —	Whole-grain, bran
Cheese	All except —	Those containing seeds or spices and very strongly flavoured cheeses
Desserts	Ice-cream, sorbet, custards, jellies, yoghurts	Those with forbidden fruits and nuts
Eggs	All except —	Fried
Fats	All except —	Fried foods
Fruit and fruit juices	All juices, avocado, banana, canned or cooked apples, apricots, cherries, grapefruit, peaches, pears, seedless grapes	All raw fruit, all dried fruit, berries, coconut, figs, grapes, melon, pineapple, plums, rhubarb
Fish and meat	Baked, boiled, roasted, and stewed beef, lamb, veal, or liver, roasted or casseroled pork, chicken, duck, turkey, cooked fish without bones — except fried	Fried, salted, and smoked meats, corned beef, sausage and cold meats, game birds, goose, fried fish, shellfish, anchovies, herrings, sardines
Milk	All	None
Potatoes, rice and pasta	Baked, boiled, mashed potatoes, dumplings, noodles, boiled rice, spaghetti	Fried potatoes or chips, potato salad, jacket potatoes, bread stuffing, chow mein, barley
Soups	Broths, consommé, bouillon, creamed, and strained vegetable	Onion, beans, pea, bisques, game, chowders
Sweets	Butterscotch, caramels, chocolate, fudge, marsh mallows, mints, honey, jelly, syrups	Candied fruits, nuts, chewing gum, jams, preserves, marmalade, marzipan, fruits

	Allowed	*Forbidden*
Vegetable	Cooked asparagus, beans, carrots, courgettes, mushrooms, spinach, tomatoes, tomato juice, and other vegetable juices	All raw vegetables, legumes
Condiments and spices	All except —	Garlic, horseradish, olives, pickled onions, chilli, relishes, meat sauces, whole herbs and spices

Low residue diet. This is often recommended during or for a while after intestinal radiotherapy. It decreases the amount of fibre or roughage and reduces other foods (milk products) that may irritate the bowel and cause diarrhoea.

	Allowed	*Forbidden*
Drinks	All	Limit milk to 2 cups per day
Bread and cereal	All except —	Whole-grain levels and cereals, bran, breads containing nuts and raisins
Flour	All except —	Whole-grain, bran
Cheese	Cottage and cream cheese, other mild cheeses (1 oz substituted for 1 cup milk)	All others
Desserts	Custards, jellies, plain cakes and biscuits, sorbets	All desserts containing seeds, nuts, raisins, and coconut. Fruits with a tough skin
Eggs	All except —	Fried
Fats	All except —	Tartar sauce, salad dressing containing seeds
Fruit and fruit juices	All juices, canned, or cooked fruit, peeled fruit without seeds, apples, apricots, avocados, bananas, cherries, grapefruit, oranges, tangerines, grapes, melons, peaches, pears, pineapples, and plums	All other fresh fruits, dried fruits, berries, figs
Fish and meat	Well cooked beef, lamb, veal, liver, poultry and ham — baked, stewed, and roasted. Fresh or frozen fish without bones, canned salmon, or tuna	Fried meats, smoked, cured and cold meats, corned beef, and sausage. All fried or smoked fish, sardine, and herring
Vegetables	Asparagus, beans, carrots, mushrooms, peas, spinach, tomatoes, turnips, tomato juice, lettuce	All raw vegetables except lettuce, dried peas or beans, nuts and any cereal or cooked vegetables
Milk and milk products	Milk and skimmed milk to 2 cups per day. Yoghurt	Yoghurt containing forbidden fruits

	Allowed	*Forbidden*
Potatoes, rice and pasta	Mashed, scalloped baked potatoes without skin. Boiled white rice, macaroni, noodles, spaghetti	Fried potatoes, potato salad, brown rice
Soups	Cream soups and broths made with allowed foods	All others
Condiments and spices	Ground or finely chopped herbs and spices, salt, flavouring extract, ketchup, gravy, white sauces, vinegar, soy sauce	Olives, pickles, chilli, all other spices

High fibre diet. This is used to increase the amount of roughage (fibre) in the diet so that the increased bulk in the intestine stimulates the bowel. The diet can be useful when constipation is caused by drugs or inactivity. The diet is essentially normal but includes two or three meals with foods high in bulk and roughage; suggested foods include:

Bread and cereals	: Use whole-grain cereals such as bran and shredded wheat. Bread should be whole-grain.
Potatoes, rice, and pasta	: Use potatoes, brown rice, and whole-grain pasta rather than refined products.
Vegetables	: Include salad and raw vegetables.
Fruit	: Eat whole fruits and skins, stewed and dried fruits, and juices, figs, raisins, and nuts.

Other helpful books

General reference source for publication

Coping with Cancer: an Annotated Bibliography (1980)

U.S. Department of Health Education and Welfare,
Public Health Service,
National Cancer Institute,
Bethesda,
Maryland 20205,
USA

General books

Conquering Cancer (1981)

Israel,
Pelican

Cancer: the Facts (1980)

Sir Ronald Bodley Scott,
Oxford University Press

Coping with Cancer (1980)

U.S. Department of Health, and Human Services,
National Cancer Institute,
Bethesda,
Maryland 20205,
USA

Cancer Care: A Personal Guide (1979)

Harold Glucksberg and Jack Singer,
The Johns Hopkins University Press,
Baltimore,
USA

You Can Fight Cancer and Win (1977)

J. Brody and A. Hollets,
Times Books Inc.,
New York,
N.Y. 10016,
USA

Specific tumours

You and Leukaemia: A Day at a Time (1978)
(specifically for children)

Lynn Baker,
W.B. Saunders Co.

Breast Cancer: The Facts (1981)

Michael Baum,
Oxford University Press

The Breast Cancer Digest (1980)

U.S. Department of Health, and Human Services,
National Cancer Institute,
Bethesda,
Maryland 20205,
USA

What Every Woman Should Know About Breast Cancer (1976)

J. Newman,
Major Books,
Canoga Park,
Ca. 91304,
USA

Your Breast and Its Care (1976)

T. Shantha,
Frederick Fells Inc.,
New York,
N.Y. 10016,
USA

A Book for Parents of Children with Leukaemia (1975)

E. Johnson and M. Miller,
Hawthorn Books Inc.,
New York,
N.Y. 10016,
USA

Living with Lung Cancer: a Reference Book for People with Lung Cancer and Their Families (1977)

B. Cox, D. Carr, and R. Lee,
Schmidt Printing Inc.,
Rochester,
MN 55901,
USA

Living with a Colostomy (1981)

Margaret Schindler,
Thorus Publishers Ltd.,
Wellingborough

Breast Cancer (1979)

Carolyn Foulder,
Pan Books,
London

Children with Cancer: a Handbook for Families and Helpers (1979)

M. Parker,
Callell

See various associations (page 352) for leaflets on individual tumours.

Prevention

Preventing Cancer: What You Can Do To Cut Your Risks by up to 50% (1978)

Elizabeth Whelan,
Sphere Books Ltd.,
London

Talking about cancer

Taking time

U.S. Department of Health and Human Services,
National Cancer Institute,
Bethesda,
Maryland 20205,
USA

Where can the cancer patient and their family get help?

BRITAIN

C.A.R.E. Cancer Aftercare and Rehabilitation Society

> Sec. G.W. Poole,
> Lodge Cottage,
> Church Lane,
> Timbsbury, Bath
>
> Telephone: 0761–70731.

A self-help group of ex-cancer patients and their friends who help cancer patients to return to a normal life. Branches have been formed in Hastings, Huddersfield, London, Worthing, and Edinburgh.

Cancer Research Campaign

> 2 Carlton House Terrace,
> London SW1Y 9AR
>
> Telephone: 01–930–8972.

Supports cancer research and cancer units in various parts of the country. Has over 900 local branches throughout the country. Main aim is to promote research.

Colostomy Welfare Group

38–39 Eccleston Square,
London SW1V 1PB.

Telephone: 01-828-5175.

Aims to help the mental, physical, and spiritual adjustment of those who have had or are about to have a colostomy. All officers of the association have colostomies and can give advice from personal experience. Home and hospital visiting is an important aspect of their work. This group has branches in various parts of the country.

CRUSE – The national organization for the widowed and their children

Cruse House,
126 Sheen Road,
Richmond,
Surrey TW9 1UR

Telephone: 01-940-4818 (9047)

Offers a counselling service to help with the emotional difficulties of bereavement. A network of local branches exists throughout the country.

Ileostomy Association of Great Britain and Ireland

Central Office,
1st Floor,
23 Winchester Road,
Basingstoke RG21 1UE

Telephone: 0256-21288

A mutual aid association for those with a permanent ileostomy. Their main object is to help people with an ileostomy resume a full life as soon as possible. They will visit patients in their home or hospital. There are over 50 divisions throughout the country.

Imperial Cancer Research Fund

P.O. Box 123,
Lincoln's Inn Fields,
London WC2A 3PX

Telephone: 01-242 0200

This organization is concerned with cancer research and in addition to running two large research centres funds projects in other hospitals and laboratories.

Leukaemia Research Fund

43 Great Ormond Street,
London WC1N 3JJ

Telephone: 01-405 0101

Exists to encourage, promote, and assist research into leukaemia and similar blood disorders. Supports research in over 40 centres in Britain. There are 160 local branches throughout the country. Does publish some information leaflets for patients with lymphomas and leukaemias.

The Leukaemia Society

186 Torbay Road,
Rayners Lane,
Harrow,
Middlesex HA2 9QL

Telephone: 01-868 4107

The society was formed by parents, some of whom had leukaemic children, with the object of helping others in the same position. Membership is now open to adult sufferers and their families. Help is available in different parts of Britain.

Malcolm Sargent Cancer Fund for Children

Administrative Office,
6 Sydney Street,
London SW3 6PP

Telephone: 01-352 6884

Exists to give financial aid and support to children suffering from cancer and their families, either in their own homes or in hospital. An application for a grant is made by the GP, social worker, or district nurse and money is available for a wide range of needs. In addition to individual grants the fund maintains its own social workers in Belfast, Birmingham, Edinburgh, Liverpool, London, Manchester, and Newcastle.

Marie Curie Fund

Head Office,
28 Belgrave Square,
London SW1X 8QG

Telephone: 01-235 3325

The foundation is mainly concerned with providing skilled nursing care to cancer patients. This is available through eleven residential nursing homes and a nationwide home nursing service.

The Mastectomy Association

25 Brighton Road,
South Croydon,
Surrey,
CR2 6EA

Telephone: 01-654 8643

This association is a group of women who have had a mastectomy and who are willing to talk with, and reassure other women who have recently had a breast removed. The association is nationwide but is centrally organized.

National Association of Laryngectomy Clubs

39 Eccleston Square,
London SW1V 1PB

Telephone: 01-834 2857

The basic aim of the laryngectomy club is to give patients the opportunity to meet and practice speaking in a sympathetic environment. It also gives support for those about to undergo an operation or those who are recovering from surgery.

National Society for Cancer Relief

Michael Sobell House,
30 Dorset Square,
London NW1 6QL

Telephone: 01-402 8125

The main object is to give practical help to cancer sufferers in need. Much of this assistance takes a financial form. Special grants are given to help pay heavy debts, fuel bills, nursing and convalescent home fees, day and night nursing, fares for treatment and relatives for visiting. Application is made via the hospital social work service, social services departments, and community nursing services. They also support a number of Macmillan continuing care units and their home care services.

Stoma Advisory Service

Abbott Laboratories Ltd.,
Queenborough,
Kent

Telephone: 07956-3371

Although run by a manufacturer this group will provide independent advice and publishes useful booklets.

Tenovus Cancer Information Centre

College Building,
University Place,
Splott,
Cardiff CF1 1SA

Telephone: 0222-483500

This centre was set up to inform the public about cancer. It is associated with Tenovus, a group supporting cancer research.

The Compassionate Friends

25 Kingsdown Parade,
Bristol B56 5UE

Telephone: 0272-47316

This is an organization of bereaved parents who through their own experience offer help to other bereaved parents.

The Urinary Conduit Association

c/o L. Kennifick,
Christie Hospital and Holt Radium Institute,
Wilmslow Road,
Withington,
Manchester 20

Provides information for patients who have had a urinary diversion.

Wessex Cancer Trust

Royal South Hants Hospital,
Graham Road,
Southampton SO9 4PE

Telephone: 0703-34288 (Ext 447/448)

An independent charity established to raise money for cancer care and research in the Wessex region. It operates as an 'umbrella' organization for the region, promoting research, care of cancer sufferers as well as public education.

Women's National Cancer Control Campaign

1 South Audley Street,
London W1Y 5DQ

Telephone: 01-499 7532/4

This group promotes measures for the early detection of cancers of the cervix and breast by health education and screening programmes.

UNITED STATES OF AMERICA

Many of these groups can provide direct help, but if not they will be able to identify where help is available. There are increasing numbers of organizations to help cancer patients and this list cannot be exhaustive but includes most of the large ones.

The American Cancer Society

Main Office: 777 Third Avenue,
New York,
New York 10017

Telephone: (212) 371-2900

This large organization provides many services which vary from city to city. They have about 3000 local centres and they will have a listing in the telephone directory of most communities. The central office in New York can advise on what facilities are available in each locality. Their main functions are:

Transportation to and from hospital or your doctor's office.
Cancer detection programmes.
Cancer education.
Supply of equipment such as special beds, couches, etc.
Nursing and home-making services.
Rehabilitation programmes.
Ostomy advice.

Cancer Care Inc. of the National Cancer Foundation

Cancer Care Inc.,
One Park Avenue,
New York,
New York 10016

Telephone: (212) 679-5700

A voluntary social service agency providing professional counselling and planning to patients with advanced cancer and their
families. Planning may include help with nursing care and
housekeeping facilities. Services are provided mainly for New
York, New Jersey, and Connecticut.

Candlelighters

Candlelighters Foundation,
123 C Street, SE,
Washington DC 20003

Telephone: (202) 483-9100 or (202) 544-1696

This is a national organization of groups for parents of children
with cancer. There are groups in most States although not all are
called Candlelighters. Their aims include:

Exchange of practical information.
Informal self-help sessions.
Information on sources of professional counselling.

Can Surmount (a programme of the American Cancer Society)

American Cancer Society,
777 Third Avenue,
New York,
New York 10017

Telephone: (212) 371-2900

This programme aims to provide volunteer support to cancer
patients and their families. After referral from the patient's doctor
a trained volunteer, who is also a cancer patient will contact
patients and their family.

360

I Can Cope (a programme of the American Cancer Society)

> American Cancer Society,
> 777 Third Avenue,
> New York,
> New York 10017
>
> Telephone: (212) 371-2900

An educational and psychological support programme developed in the North Memorial Medical Center, Minneapolis, Minnesota. The course consists of a series of classes taught by health professionals.

Leukaemia Society of America Inc.

> Leukaemia Society of America Inc.
> 211 East 42nd Street,
> New York,
> New York 10017
>
> Telephone: (212) 573-8484

Provides financial assistance and information support to patients with leukaemia, lymphoma, or Hodgkin's disease.

Make Today Count

> Make Today Count,
> P.O. Box 303,
> Burlington,
> Iowa 52601
>
> Telephone: (319) 754-7266 or (319) 754-8977.

This is a self-help group of people with incurable illnesses (including cancer), their families, nurses, physicians, and other health care professionals. Their aim is to bring together seriously ill people in order to discuss and resolve personal and emotional problems.

The National Hospice Organization

The National Hospice Organization,
Tower Suite 506,
301 Maple Avenue West,
Vienna, Virginia 22180

This is an organization that can give information on hospices (see (page 317) in the United States.

United Cancer Council Inc.

United Cancer Council Inc.,
1803 N. Meridian Street,
Indianapolis,
Indiana 46202

Telephone: (317) 923-6490

This is a federation of voluntary cancer agencies, who seek to control cancer by a programme of service, education, and research. They will provide help with:

Screening programmes,
Rehabilitation services,
Nursing, drugs, and house-keeping services,
Health education.

United Ostomy Association

United Ostomy Association Inc.,
111 Wilshire Boulevard,
Los Angeles,
California 90017

Telephone: (213) 481-2811

An association which offers emotional and practical support to patients with ostomies (page 326).

The Cancer Information Service

This is a service provided by the National Cancer Institute. It is a toll-fee telephone enquiry system that provides information about cancer and available resources. The telephone listing (by State) is as follows:

Alabama	1–800–292–6201	Massachusetts	1–800–952–7420
Alaska	1–800–683–6070	Minnesota	1–800–582–5262
California	1–800–252–9066	Montana	1–800–525–0231
(from 213, 714, and 805)		New Hampshire	1–800–225–7034
Colorado	1–800–322–1850	New Jersey	
Connecticut	1–800–922–0824	(Northern)	800–223–1000
Delaware	1–800–523–3586	(Southern)	800–523–3586
District of		New Mexico	1–800–525–0231
Columbia	(202) 636–5700	New York City	(212) 794–7982
(including surburban Maryland		New York State	1–800–462–7255
and northern Virginia)		North Carolina	1–800–672–0943
Florida	1–800–432–5953	North Dakota	1–800–328–5188
Georgia	1–800–327–7332	Ohio	1–800–282–6522
Hawaii		Pennsylvania	1–800–822–3963
Oahu	524–1234	South Dakota	1–800–328–5188
Other islands		Texas	1–800–392–2040
ask operator for	Enterprise 6702	Vermont	1–800–225–7034
Illinois	800–972–0586	Washington	1–800–552–7212
Kentucky	800–432–9321	Wisconsin	1–800–362–8038
Maine	1–800–225–7034	Wyoming	1–800–525–0231
Maryland	800–492–1444	All other areas	800–638–6694

AUSTRALIA

Individual societies and groups caring for patients with particular tumours can be contacted through the relevant cancer societies.

Australian Cancer Society

Box 4708,
Sydney, NSW 2001

Telephone: (02) 231-3355

Act Cancer Society

Dr. W. Burch,
Acting Chairman,
Department of Nuclear Medicine,
Royal Canberra Hospital,
Acton, ACT 2601

Telephone: 4321-11

Dr J. Cossey,
Secretary,
Department of Pure Maths,
The Faculties,
Australian National University,
Canberra, ACT 2601

Telephone: 49-3625

Anti-cancer Council of the Queensland Cancer Fund

Mr W.L. Rudder,
Secretary,
P.O. Box 201,
North Brisbane, Qld 4000

Telephone: (07) 229-7077

Anti-cancer Council of Victoria

Miss Adrienne J. Holzer,
90 Jolimont Street,
East Melbourne, Vic 3002

Telephone: (03) 654-2411

Anti-cancer Foundation of the Universities of South Australia

Mr T.R. Osborn,
Executive Secretary,
GPO Box 498,
Adelaide, SA 5001

Telephone: (08) 228-5027 or 5333

Cancer Council of Western Australia

Mr C. Deverall,
705 Murray Street,
West Perth, WA 6005

Telephone: (09) 321-6224 or 2365

New South Wales State Cancer Council

Mr R. Williams,
Secretary,
GPO Box 7070,
Sydney, NSW 2001

Telephone: (02) 233-2300

Tasmanian Cancer Committee

Mr L.J. Baillie,
Secretary/Treasurer,
c/o Health Services Department,
GPO Box 191B,
Hobart, TAS 7001

Telephone: (022) 30-3262

Northern Territory Anti-cancer Foundation

Mrs L. Finch,
Secretary,
GPO Box 718,
Darwin, NT 5790

Telephone: (089) 81-8415 or 3556

CANADA

Individual societies and groups caring for patients with particular tumours can be contacted through the relevant cancer societies.

Canadian Cancer Society

National Office,
Suite 1001,
130 Bloor Street West,
Toronto,
Ontario M5S 2V5

Telephone: 416-961-7223

British Colombia and Yukon

Mrs Phillis Hood,
Executive Director,
Canadian Cancer Society,
955 West Broadway,
Vancouver, BC V5Z 3XB

Telephone: 604-736-1211

Alberta

Mr Tom Steele,
Executive Director,
Canadian Cancer Society,
Main Floor,
1134 – 8th Avenue S.W.,
Calgary, Alberta T2P 1J5

Telephone: 403-263-3120

Saskatchewan

Mr Roger Freeman,
Executive Director,
Canadian Cancer Society,
2629 – 29th Avenue,
Regina, Saskatchewan S4S 2Y9

Telephone: 306-525-5817

Manitoba

Mr Murray Bater,
Executive Director,
Canadian Cancer Society,
777 Portage Avenue, 2nd Floor,
Winnipeg, Manitoba R3G 0N3

Telephone: 204-774-7483

Ontario

Mr Harry Rowlands,
Executive Director,
Canadian Cancer Society,
185 Bloor Street East,
Toronto, Ontario M4W 3G5

Telephone: 416-923-7474

Quebec

Mr Guy Angers,
Executive Director,
Canadian Cancer Society,
1118 St Catherine St. W., Ste. 700,
Montreal, Quebec H3B 1H5

Telephone: 514-866-1112

New Brunswick

Mr C.F.A. Graham,
Executive Director,
Canadian Cancer Society,
(61 Union Street E2L 1A3 – Parcels)
PO Box 2089,
Saint John, New Brunswick E2L 3T5

Telephone: 506-652-7600

Nova Scotia

Mr Alf Joergensen, APR,
Canadian Cancer Society,
PO Box 3635 South,
Halifax, Nova Scotia B3J 3K6

Telephone: 902-423-6183

Prince Edward Island

Mr Jim Cox,
Executive Director,
Canadian Cancer Society,
57 Queen Street, 4th Floor,
PO Box 115, Hyndman Building,
Charlottetown, PE1 C1A 7K2

Telephone: 902-894-9675

Newfoundland

Mr Harry Lake,
Executive Director,
Canadian Cancer Society,
(Pippy Place – Parcels)
PO Box 8921,
St John's, Newfoundland A1B 3R9

Telephone: 709-753-6520

NEW ZEALAND

Individual societies and groups caring for patients with particular tumours can be contacted through the relevant cancer societies.

Cancer Society of New Zealand

The Secretary,
Box 10340,
Wellington

Auckland Division

PO Box 1724,
Auckland

Telephone: 540023

Waikato/Bay of Plenty Division

PO Box 134,
Hamilton

Telephone: 80683

Central Districts Division

PO Box 142,
Palmerston North

Telephone: 70911

Wellington Division

PO Box 11–125,
Wellington

Telephone: 726876

Canterbury/Westland Division

PO Box 373,
Christchurch

Telephone: 65864

Otago/Southland Division

PO Box 1245,
Dunedin

Telephone: 777042

Glossary

TECHNICAL TERMS EXPLAINED

Ablative therapy
A treatment to totally remove or eradicate part of the body.

Adenocarcinoma
A cancer starting in glandular tissue.

Adjuvant therapy
A secondary treatment which usually follows surgery and involves chemotherapy or radiotherapy.

Adjuvant treatment
The use of treatment (usually chemotherapy) after a cancer has been completely removed. This is done when there is a high chance that the cancer will return because microscopic collections of cells have spread to other parts of the body.

Adrenalectomy
Removal of the adrenal glands.

Aetiology
The study of the cause of a disease.

Alopecia
Loss of hair which can be caused by some types of chemotherapy and radiation to the scalp. It is nearly always temporary.

Amenorrhoea
Loss of normal menstruation.

Anaemia
Lack of red cells in the blood which causes tiredness, shortness of breath, and pallor.

Analgesic
Medicine given (by mouth, injection, or suppository) to control pain.

Androgen
A male hormone.

Aspirate
To suck off fluid with a syringe.

Astrocytoma
The commonest cancer that develops in the brain in adults.

Axilla
The arm pit.

Benign
A term used to describe a tumour or tissue which is not malignant or cancerous and which, therefore, does not spread.

Bilateral
Pertaining to both sides.

Biopsy (page 65)
The surgical removal of a piece of tissue for examination under a microscope.

Blood count
A test measuring the number of red cells, white cells, and platelets there are in a blood sample.

Bone marrow
Spongy tissue in the middle of bones that makes blood cells.

Bone marrow biopsy and aspiration (page 66)
The removal of a small amount of bone marrow for examination under a microscope. This is done by pushing a fine needle (after local anaesthetic) into the pelvis or the breast bone.

Brain scan (page 65)
Way of examining the brain after injecting a small amount of a radioactive 'dye'.

BSE
Breast self-examination (page 26)

Bronchoscopy (page 77)
Examination of the air passages with a flexible instrument called a bronchoscope.

Cancer
A general term for more than 100 diseases where there is uncontrolled growth of cells which spread and, if untreated, eventually leads to death.

Carcinogen
A substance that can cause or help cause cancer.

Carcinoma
A cancer that develops from cells called epithelial cells. These cells are present in the skin, lungs, glands, gastrointestinal tract, and urinary tract. Cancers that develop in these sites are called carcinomas and are the commonest type of cancer.

CAT scan (page 59)
A computerized x-ray system that gives very detailed pictures.

Chemotherapy (Chapter Fourteen)
The use of drugs to treat cancer.

Cervix
Neck of the uterus or womb.

Cervical smear *See* Pap smear.

Cobalt therapy
Radiotherapy (Chapter Thirteen) using radiation from a cobalt machine.

Colonoscopy (page 73)
The use of a flexible instrument to examine the entire large bowel.

Colostomy (page 326)
An operation to bring the bowel (colon) up to the abdominal wall so that stool may be collected in a special bag.

Colposcopy
Examination of the neck of the womb with a magnifying instrument passed into the vagina.

Combination chemotherapy (Chapter Fourteen)
The use of several drugs given together to treat cancer.

Combined modality treatment
The use of more than one type of anti-cancer treatment (surgery, radiotherapy, and chemotherapy) together.

Craniopharyngioma
A tumour of the pituitary gland at the base of the brain.

CT scan *See* CAT scan.

Cyst
A closed cavity or sac that contains liquid or semi-solid material.

Cystoscopy (page 176)
Use of an instrument passed through the passage from the bladder to examine the inside of the bladder.

DNA
The genetic material in the centre of a cell which controls its growth, division, and function.

Dysuria
Pain on passing urine.

Endocrine gland
Glands that secrete hormones into the bloodstream.

Endocrine therapy
The use of hormones to treat a disease.

Endometrium
Lining of the womb that is shed with each period.

Endoscopy
The use of a hollow instrument to examine the inside of different parts of the body.

Epidemiology
The study of the geographic distribution of disease.

Excisional biopsy
Total surgical removal of tissue to be examined.

Fibrocystic disease
A *benign* breast condition in which there is overgrowth of fibrous tissue often combined with formation of cysts.

Frozen section
A rapid way of examining a biopsy to see if it contains cancer; a result is available straightaway so that a suitable operation can be planned.

Gastroscopy (page 74)
The use of a flexible instrument, which is swallowed, to examine the inside of the stomach and upper part of the small bowel.

Genetic
Inherited.

Glioblastoma
A highly malignant brain cancer in adults.

Granulocytes (neutrophils)
Infection fighting cells in the blood.

Gynaeocolgist
A doctor who specializes in the treatment of diseases of the female reproductive tract.

Haematologist
A doctor who specializes in diseases of the blood and bone marrow.

Haematuria
Blood in the urine.

Hepatoma
A primary cancer of the liver.

Histology
The study of tissues to diagnose disease.

Hormone
A chemical substance that circulates in the blood and causes changes in the body.

Hormone therapy
The use of hormones to treat a disease.

Hormone receptor assay
A special test to see if a tumour contains special receptor sites that indicate that it is likely to respond to hormonal therapy.

Hyperalimentation
The infusion (drip) of highly nutritious fluids containing protein and lots of calories into a vein.

Hypernephroma (page 170)
A cancer of the kidney in adults.

Hypophysectomy
Surgical removal of the pituitary gland.

Hysterectomy
An operation to remove the womb (uterus).

Ileostomy
An artificial opening between the small bowel (ileum) and the abdominal wall so that stool can be collected in a bag.

Immunotherapy
An experimental method of treatment that attempts to increase the body's own defence (immune) mechanisms against cancer.

Incidence
The rate at which a certain event occurs, such as the number of new cases of cancer occurring during a certain period.

Incisional biopsy
Surgical removal of part of a tissue to be examined.

In situ cancer
The earliest stage of a cancer where it is localized just where it started.

Intravenous (IV)
Infusion of fluid into a vein.

Irradiation
Treatment by radiation.

Laparotomy
An exploratory abdominal operation.

Laryngectomy
Surgical removal of the voice box (larynx).

Laryngoscopy
Examination of the back of the throat and voice box (larynx) using a mirror.

Larynx
Voice box situated in the upper part of the wind pipe.

Lesion
Any abnormal area (for whatever reason) in a tissue.

Linear accelerator
A type of radiotherapy machine producing a very high energy radiation.

Local recurrence
A tumour that reappears at the site of the original tumour.

Localized cancer
A cancer confined to the site of origin.

Lumbar puncture (page 56)
A test examining the fluid in the spine (CSF). After the area has been injected with local anaesthetic a needle is inserted into the spine and fluid is taken out.

Lumpectomy
Surgical removal of a cancerous lump and a portion of surrounding tissue instead of the whole organ.

Lymphatic system
Circulatory network of lymph-carrying vessels, the lymph nodes, spleen, and thymus which produce and store infection-fighting cells.

Lymph nodes (glands)
Nodules of tissue in the lymphatics that make lymphocytes and filter out unwanted substances.

Lymphangiogram (page 51)
A special x-ray test to outline the lymph glands deep in the abdomen. A contrast dye is injected into the fine lymphatic vessels in the feet and this spreads to the abdomen.

Lymphocytes
White cells in the blood that produce antibodies to fight infections.

Lymphoedema
Swelling of a part of the body because the normal lymphatics have been blocked or destroyed.

Lymphoma (page 202)
A cancer that develops in the lymph system.

Malignant
A tumour which is cancerous and will spread with fatal results if not removed.

Mammogram (page 44)
A special x-ray used to detect small breast cancers.

Mastectomy (page 136)
An operation to surgically remove a breast for cancer.

Medical oncology
The treatment of cancer with drugs (chemotherapy).

Mediastinum
The area of the chest containing the heart and major blood vessels.

Mega voltage radiotherapy (Chapter Thirteen)
High energy irradiation using cobalt or linear accelerator sources.

Melanoma (page 238)
A cancer of the skin that developes from a mole.

Menarche
The beginning of menstruation at puberty.

Menopause
The cessation of menstruation.

Mesothelioma
A tumour of the lining of the lung (pleura) or of the abdomen (peritoneum) that is usually caused by asbestos.

Metastasis
The spread of a cancer from one part of the body to another. The new area of cancer is a metastasis or secondary.

Morbidity
The symptoms or effects of a disease or its treatment.

Mortality rate
The death rate.

Mucositis
Inflammation or soreness of the lining of the mouth (mucosa).

Multicentric
Having more than one centre of origin.

Mutation
A permanent change in the genetic material (DNA).

Neutrophils (granulocytes) infection fighting cells.

Neoplasm
A 'jargon word' sometimes used instead of cancer – means new growth.

Node
A lymph node.

Occult tumour
A concealed or hidden tumour.

Oncology
The study of tumours (benign and malignant).

Oophectomy (ovariectomy)
An operation to surgically remove the ovaries.

Orthovoltage radiotherapy (Chapter Thirteen)
Low energy radiation now only used to treat superficial cancers.

Ostomy (page 326)
An artificial opening between an organ and the surface of the abdominal wall. This is done so that the excretion of the intestine (colostomy or ileostomy) or urine can be collected in a bag.

Paget's disease
A cancer of the nipple.

Palliative treatment
Treatment aimed to make a person feel better rather than to cure them.

Palpate
Feel by hand.

Pap (cervical) smear (page 40)
A scraping of cells from the neck of the womb (cervix) for examination under a microscope.

Paralytic ileus
Stoppage of the bowel caused by loss of normal intestinal movement.

Pathology
The branch of medicine concerned with the examination of diseased tissues.

Pectoralis muscles
The group of muscles on the front of the chest underlying the breast.

Peritoneum
The inner lining of the abdomen.

Pituitary gland
The endocrine gland at the base of the brain which controls many other endocrine glands.

Placebo
An inert substance used in controlled trials to see if a treatment is better than no treatment at all (placebo).

Platelets
Cells in the blood that help it to clot.

Pleura
The lining over the lungs.

Polyp
A benign outgrowth of tissue.

Premalignant
An abnormal area in the body that may develop into a cancer but has not, as yet, done so.

Prevalence
The total number of cases at one time in a given area.

Primary cancer
A cancer present at the site in which it developed.

Progesterone
A hormone produced by the adrenal gland.

Prognosis
A prediction of the likely course of a disease. This can only be estimated from the experiences of a lot of patients and cannot accurately predict the outcome in an individual.

Prolactin
A pituitary hormone that stimulates milk production.

Prophylactic
Treatment designed to prevent a disease.

Prosthesis
A specially manufactured replacement to functionally and cosmetically take the place of a part of the body that has been surgically removed. The most common are artificial limbs and artificial breasts after mastectomy.

Radiation or radiotherapy (Chapter Thirteen)
A way of damaging or killing cancer cells by using a beam of radiation.

Radiation therapist (radiotherapist)
A doctor specializing in the treatment of cancer with radiation.

Radical mastectomy (Halsted)
An extensive mastectomy that includes removal of some of the muscles on the chest wall.

Radioactive implants (page 9)
The placing (implanting) of a radioactive source in the body. This is put close by a cancer and gives it a very high dose of radiation and is then removed.

Radioresistant
A tumour that does not shrink when treated with doses of radiation that can be tolerated by surrounding tissues.

Radiosensitive
A cancer that shrinks or can be eradicated by a dose of radiation that is tolerated by nearby tissues.

Reconstructive mammaplasty
The rebuilding of a breast by plastic surgery.

Relapse (recurrence) (page 288)
The regrowth of a cancer after it has been removed or has responded to treatment.

Remission (page 288)
Shrinkage of a tumour. This may be partial or complete, but does not necessarily indicate cure.

Sarcoma
Cancers that develop in the body's supporting tissues (bone, cartilage, muscle, fat, tendons) and the tissue between organs.

Side-effects
Unwanted and sometimes unpleasant reactions to treatment that are usually temporary though some may be permanent.

Sigmoidoscopy (page 72)
A visual examination of the rectum and last part of the large bowel using a straight metal tube called a sigmoidoscope.

Simple mastectomy (total mastectomy)
Surgical removal of the breast tissue only.

Staging
The systematic investigation of the extent of spread of tumour in order to decide what treatment is best. The amount of tumour spread is described as the disease stage.

Steroids
A group of naturally occurring compounds that may act as hormones.

Stomatitis
Inflammation or soreness of the mouth.

Subcutaneous mastectomy
Surgical removal of the internal breast tissue, leaving the skin and nipple used as a prophylactic measure.

Supraclavicular
The area above the clavical (collar bone). Usually used to refer to lymph nodes at this site.

Systemic
Refers to the whole body, hence systemic treatment treats the whole body.

Tyelectomy (lumpectomy)
Surgical removal of a lump with a portion of surrounding tissue instead of the whole organ.

Therapy
A treatment for a disease.

Tomograms (page 57)
Special x-rays taken to find small abnormalities.

Toxicity
The side-effects of a treatment.

Tumour
A swelling or mass of tissue in any part of the body. It may be cancerous or benign.

Ulcer
An erosion in a surface membrane (such as in the stomach) that may be benign or malignant.

Ultrasound test (ultrasonography) (page 59)
The use of a very high frequency sound (which the ear cannot hear) to look inside the body.

Xeroradiograph
A special x-ray of the breast.

Index